Feil/Lippert/Lozac'h/Palazzini/Amaral
Atlas of Surgical Stapling

Atlas of Surgical Stapling

Edited by

W. Feil, H. Lippert, P. Lozac'h, G. Palazzini, J. Amaral

With Contributions by

B. Descottes, W. Feil, T. Fullem, G. B. Grassi, H. Lippert, A. Longo, P. Lozac'h, M. Martelli, G. Palazzini, J. Sökeland, P. H. Sugarbaker

Editorial Advisors:

K. Haas, A. Ruhalter

Editorial Assistance:

Elizabeth Chamberlain

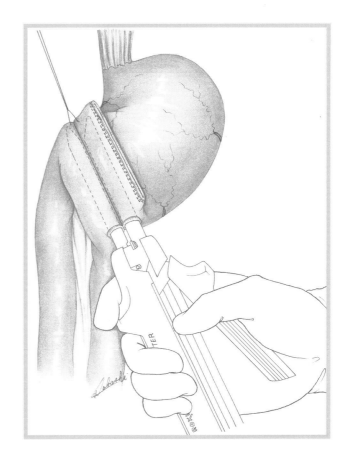

 Johann Ambrosius Barth · Heidelberg

Contributors

Italy: Prof. Dr. G.B. Grassi (Rome)
            Dr. A. Longo (Palermo)
            Prof. Dr. M. Martelli (Rome)
            Prof. Dr. G. Palazzini (Rome)

France: Prof. Dr. B. Descottes (Limoges)
            Prof. Dr. P. Lozac'h (Brest)

Germany: Prof. Dr. H. Lippert (Magdeburg)
            Prof. Dr. J. Sökeland (Dortmund)

Austria: Prof. Dr. W. Feil (Vienna)

USA: Joe Amaral, M.D., F.A.C.S.
            Terrence Fullem, M.D., F.A.C.S.
            Paul H. Sugarbaker, M.D., F.A.C.S.

            Editorial Advisors:
            Kara Haas, M.D., F.A.C.S.
            Aaron Ruhalter, M.D., F.A.C.S.

            Editorial Assistance:
            Elizabeth Chamberlain

Typesetting: Ch. Molter, Heidelberg, Germany
Cover Design: Wachter Design, Schwetzingen, Germany
Printing and Binding: Kösel, Kempten, Germany

ISBN 3-8304-5069-9

Preface

Aims of the Atlas of Surgical Stapling

The main objective of this book is to serve as a guide to the application of mechanical staplers and other surgical devices in different surgical procedures.

The first section covers the history of stapling and describes the various staplers, other technological aids, and basic stapling techniques in sufficient detail to provide the reader with a broad understanding of the principles of surgical stapling.

In the second section, the authors describe the application of mechanical staplers and other surgical devices according to their individual surgical expertise and school of thought, which may differ from the opinions of other, equally valid schools or surgical practices.

The ultimate aim of this book is to give the surgeon a better understanding of, and insight into, the use of mechanical staplers and other devices in daily practice, thus enhancing surgery and improving patient care.

Contents

I Mechanical Stapling and other Surgical Devices

II Surgical Procedures

1 Thoracic Surgery

2 Esophageal Surgery

3 Gastric Surgery

4 Pancreatic Surgery

5 Small Bowel Surgery

6 Large Bowel Surgery

7 Colorectal Surgery

8 Gynecological Surgery

9 Urological Surgery

III References

I

Mechanical Stapling and other Surgical Devices

1 History of Mechanical Stapling

For centuries, surgeons have been aware of the importance of providing leak-proof anastomoses and hemostatic wound closures. It was observed that another factor for success was to invert the tissue while performing a closure or an anastomosis. This has typically been achieved through the careful application of sutures. However, surgeons have more recently looked for better ways to close or anastomose tissues.

In 1826, Henroz, a surgeon from Belgium, presented a device made from two rings that allowed the surgeon to approximate everted tissues from two bowel segments. He successfully used this device on dogs. Others began to study the use of devices (Travers, Lembert, and Denans) but without paying too much attention to the inversion or eversion of tissue.

In 1892, John B. Murphy from Chicago developed an anastomotic ring (Fig. 1a, b) which was intended to be used on cholecystoduodenostomies. This device became very popular and was subsequently used for bowel and gastric anastomoses. Murphy proved that it was possible to create a mechanical device to perform an anastomosis; however, manual sutures were becoming more and more reliable and were often preferred to this type of device. Adalbert Ramaugé, a South American surgeon, also presented an anastomotic ring at about the same time, but his device never became as popular.

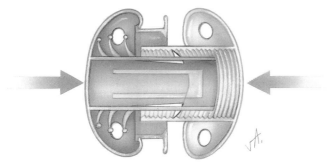

Fig. 1a Murphy ring: technical aspect

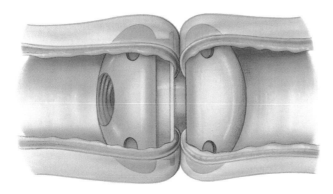

Fig. 1b Murphy ring in place

Many of the principles of mechanical stapling in surgery were defined by Humer Hültl in Budapest in 1909. The most important principles he focused upon were:

1) Tissue compression
2) Tissue stapling while using a metallic wire to form B-shaped staples
3) B-shape of the closed staple
4) Staggered positioning of two staple lines to perform the procedure

With the help of Victor Fischer, Hültl created an instrument used to close the stomach during gastrectomies (Fig. 2). The limitations of this instrument lay in its weight and bulk. In 1921 Aladar von Petz, another Hungarian surgeon, created a light and easy-to-use instrument based on the same principles as Hültl's. This instrument was more readily adopted in the surgical field, even though it did not have a double-staggered staple line (Fig. 3).

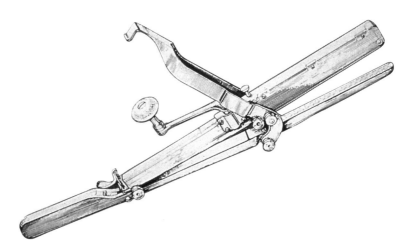

Fig. 2 Hültl stapler

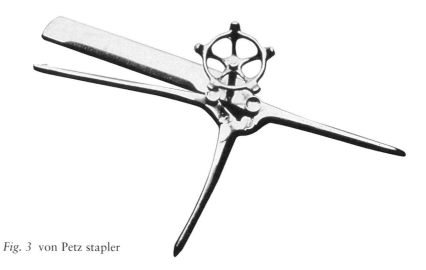

Fig. 3 von Petz stapler

Subsequently, this instrument was improved by H. Friedrich (Fig. 4) and Neuffer in Germany. The two main changes were simultaneous tissue compression and staple firing, and the creation of cartridges that allowed the instrument to be used several times during the same operation. However, the staples still were not placed in a staggered fashion. N. Nakayama from Japan further improved von Petz's instrument, but again without changing the staple position.

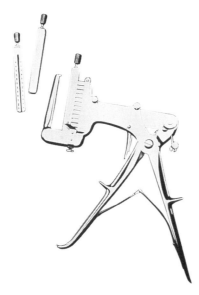

Fig. 4 Friedrich stapler

Many other instruments were developed, but they were never used as often as von Petz's. These instruments were good but not yet ideal.

The next phase of development began at the end of World War II in Moscow, USSR. The war had disastrous effects on the population. The resulting decline in the number of surgeons led to thousands of deaths.

Because hospitals and care centers were few and far between, there was a need for instruments that would allow inadequately trained surgeons to carry out standardized surgical procedures quickly in emergencies. This was the reason for the creation of the Scientific Institute for Surgical Devices and Instruments. During the 1950s, this institute developed many mechanical stapling devices that were adopted widely throughout the country. These included:

- Instruments for linear stapling, with reloadable cartridges using stainless steel staples. Many different models were built, but the principle of placing a double *linear* row of staples to approximate tubular structures remained.

- Instruments to create side-by-side anastomoses between two bowel lumens. This type of instrument allowed the placement of two double rows of staples while simultaneously cutting between these rows.
- Instruments to create end-to-end, end-to-side, or side-to-end circular anastomoses.

These instruments often needed a manually placed suture to complete the staple lines. They also required a great deal of preparation before firing as well as considerable maintenance. They were, however, reliable and consequently were used throughout the USSR.

The third phase in the development of mechanical stapling started with the visit of an American surgeon, Mark Ravitch, to Kiev. There, he observed a Russian surgeon using a mechanical stapler on a bronchus. Dr. Ravitch then worked in his laboratory in Baltimore on the complete line of Russian products and evaluated their performance. He developed a totally new series of American instruments and founded a new company that focused on surgical staplers. These products were quite different from the Russian ones:

- The staplers remained reusable, but they came with plastic, preloaded staple cartridges that were sterilized, sold in a single package, and intended for single-patient use.
- The instruments were lighter and easier to use and could deliver different lengths of staple lines.
- All the instruments, including the circular stapler, delivered a double-staggered row of staples, which was not the case with the first generation of Russian instruments.

By the 1970s the use of linear staplers, linear cutters, and circular staplers, was widespread in American hospitals throughout the world. Today, they continue to be the foundation of surgical stapling in the OR.

The fourth and latest phase in the development of mechanical staplers was the introduction of single-patient-use instruments. At the end of the 1970s, surgeons became aware of the risk of cross-contamination and cost per procedure. With the launch of the first completely disposable single-patient-use mechanical stapler by Ethicon, Inc., in 1976 (a skin stapler) (Fig. 5), other manufacturers of mechanical staplers began changing the way they manufactured their products by focusing on single-patient-use products (disposable).

While some manufacturers retained a number of reusable products in their product line, Ethicon Inc., focused exclusively on a single-patient-use option to ensure reliability, lower maintenance, and sterility of the staplers.

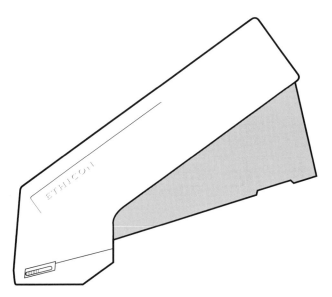

Fig. 5 Single-patient-use skin stapler

Variations of the standard instruments were then developed:

- Articulating liner staplers
- Miniaturized instruments for endoscopic use
- Automatic clip appliers

In 1989, stainless steel staples and clips were replaced with titanium. It has been demonstrated that titanium is more biocompatible, allowing for less distortion of radiologic exams (MRI, plain films, and nuclear medicine).

Another important improvement was to use absorbable materials for clips, making them radiolucent.

Recently, new adjunctive technologies have been developed to facilitate and complement the use of mechanical staplers, the most important one being the use of ultrasonic energy as a means to cut, dissect, and coagulate tissue.

2 Product Description of Mechanical Staplers and Other Surgical Devices

Principles of Surgical Stapling

The basic requirements for an anastomosis are:
– Creation of an adequate lumen
– Maintenance of adequate tissue vascularization
– Prevention of leakage and fistulas
– Avoidance of tissue tension
– Hemostasis

Staple Formation

The staples currently used in the majority of devices have a rectangular shape that changes into a B-shaped form after compression against the anvil of the stapler. This principle is shown in the figures below. The staple height refers to the distance in millimeters remaining within the staple when the staple is closed.

Because tissues to be stapled have different thicknesses, the staples need to come in different dimensions. This is to accommodate different tissues and at the same time to adhere to the surgical stapling principles mentioned above. Two technologies are available today that permit this: one delivers a predetermined staple height and the other allows variation of staple height formation.

Fixed Staple Height

Instruments using this technology deliver a closed staple with the following staple heights:

2.0 mm   1.5 mm   1.0 mm

Variable Staple Height

In this case, with one instrument the surgeon can adapt the staple height to the tissue thickness to be stapled. Instruments using this technology will deliver staple heights ranging from 2.5 mm to 1.0 mm.

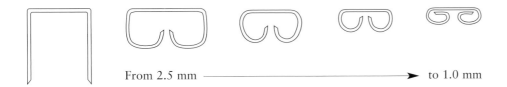

Linear Staplers

Linear staplers deliver a double-staggered row of staples. They are available with fixed or variable staple heights. Examples of applications include:

- Closure of internal organs prior to transection
- Closure of the common opening or an enterotomy
  after creation of an anastomosis
- Creation of an end-to-end anastomosis (triangulation)

Variable staple height:

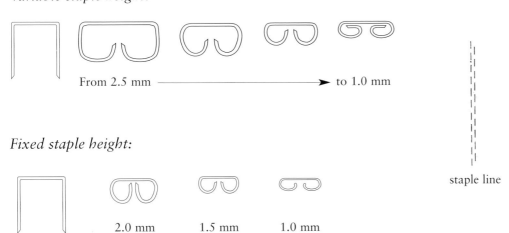

Linear Cutters

Linear cutters deliver double-staggered rows of staples while simultaneously transecting the tissue between the rows. They are available only with fixed staple heights. Applications include:

– Creating side-to-side and functional end-to-end anastomoses

– Making terminal closures

Fixed staple height:

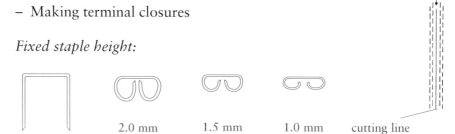

2.0 mm   1.5 mm   1.0 mm   cutting line

Circular Staplers

Circular staplers deliver two circular-staggered rows of staples, while simultaneously creating a uniform stoma between the organs to be anastomosed. They are only available with variable staple height. Applications include:

– Creating end-to-end anastomoses

– Creating end-to-side anastomoses

Variable staple height:

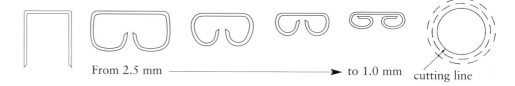

From 2.5 mm   to 1.0 mm   cutting line

Technical Aspects of Staples

Depending on the kind of instrument and the procedure, surgical staplers create inverted or everted tissue approximation. Further refinement of the surgical staplers led to material changes from silver to stainless steel to titanium, which is in use today. Compared with materials formerly used, titanium offers considerable advantages.

- Titanium is the most biocompatible material.

- Artifacts caused by titanium staples during X-ray examinations are minimal.

The characteristics of titanium with regard to imaging technology, such as MRI and CT, are more favorable:

- Titanium is not affected by static magnetic fields.

- During MRI or CT, the temperature increases in a titanium staple a maximum of 0.1°C, therefore minimizing the staple as a possible source of tissue damage.

In the course of improving the staple, its application method was also being improved. Early stapling instruments compressed the tissues excessively, and the staples were then formed under this extreme pressure. Present-generation stapling instruments offer controlled tissue compression by means of adjustable staple heights, allowing the surgeon to adjust the staple height to the corresponding tissue.

With the ability to adjust the staple height, a less traumatic application of staples can be achieved. The result is that tissue blood flow is preserved in the intramural vessels and capillaries along the staple line. This improves wound healing. The same result is achieved with fixed-staple-height instruments by selecting the appropriate stapler. During this period of development, the wire thickness of the staple was also reduced considerably. Today, the thickness is between 0.2 mm and 0.3 mm, depending on the stapling instrument. This corresponds to a suture thickness of 2-0 to 3-0.

The height of the open staple legs varies and creates a variety of staple closures, from 1.0 mm to 2.5 mm. Some devices may permit adjusting the staple closure to the exact thickness of the tissue, in order to adhere to the principles previously mentioned.

In some cases a fixed staple closure provides a good suture/anastomosis and may allow the design of more easily handled instruments.

The different staple closures currently in use are identified by different color codes:

Color Code	Fixed Staple Height			Type of Tissue
White				Vascular/Thin
Blue	2.0 mm	1.5 mm	1.0 mm	Standard
Green				Thick

	Variable Staple Height				
Grey					Standard
Yellow					Thick
	From 2.5 mm ⟶ to 1.0 mm				

Generally, the principles for surgical stapling are also valid for mechanical ligating clips. For mechanical ligation, however, it is very important that the selected clip size corresponds with the vessel caliber to be ligated (refer to clip illustration page 25, 27).

When using surgical stapling instruments it is important to realize that, as with manual surgical sutures, a learning process must take place.

Mechanical Staplers
Staple Dimensions and Applications

Vascular/Thin (white)	Standard (blue/grey)	Thick (green/yellow)

Staple Dimensions (open):

3.0 × 2.5 mm

Staple Dimensions (open):

3.0 × 3.5 or 3.85 mm

Staple Dimensions (open):

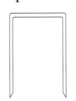

4.0 × 3.5, 4.8, or 5.5 mm

Staple Dimensions (closed):

1.0 mm

Staple Dimensions (closed):

1.5 mm

Staple Dimensions (closed):

2.0 mm

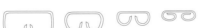

2.5 – 1.0 mm*

2.5 – 1.0 mm*

Applications

- Thin tissues
- Vascularized tissues
  (e.g., omentum, mesentery)
- Arteries and Veins

Applications

- Standard tissues
- Gastrointestinal tract
  (e.g., small bowel, esophagus)
- Lung

Applications

- Thick tissues
- Gastrointestinal tract
  (e.g., stomach)
- Bronchus/Rectum
- Lung

*Adjustable staple height

Linear Staplers

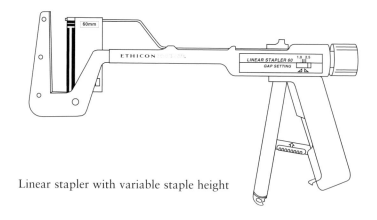

Linear stapler with variable staple height

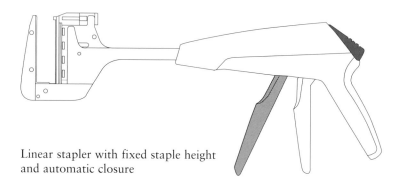

Linear stapler with fixed staple height
and automatic closure

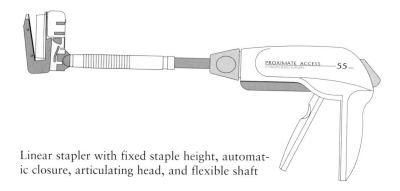

Linear stapler with fixed staple height, automatic closure, articulating head, and flexible shaft

As with all stapling instruments, linear staplers have applications in nearly all surgical procedures, especially for closure of organs, closure of incisions, ligation of large vessels, and, in rare cases, for end-to-end anastomoses.

The instruments are available in different staple sizes and different staple line lengths. They create staple lines of 30 mm, 55 mm, 60 mm, or 90 mm to accommodate different tissues. One type of instrument allows staple formation to a predefined height, the other enables variable adjustment of the staple height to the specific organ according to the tissue thickness. Furthermore, various wire diameters enable stapling of different types of tissue, e.g., vessels, bronchus, or bowel.

Linear staplers deliver a double-staggered row of staples.

(Exception: The TX model delivers a triple staggered row of staples.)

The vascular linear stapler is intended specifically for vascular structures to ligate large-caliber vessels.

Do not use linear staplers on ischemic or necrotic tissue.

Linear staplers may be reloaded during a single procedure (TX: seven times; TL, TLH, TLV: three times).

Staple Lines

30 mm Vascular Linear Stapler

three staggered rows of staples*

30 mm Linear Stapler

two staggered rows of staples

55 mm Linear Stapler

two staggered rows of staples

60 mm Linear Stapler

two staggered rows of staples

90 mm Linear Stapler

two staggered rows of staples

*Only on TX model

Articulating Linear Staplers

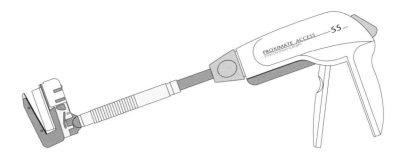

Articulating linear staplers have been designed to facilitate access in narrowed areas; therefore, the working end of the instrument can be adjusted to the site.

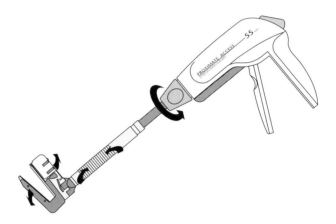

The articulating linear stapler has a 55-mm staple line and is available for standard or thick tissue. It should be noted that articulating linear staplers are not reloadable.

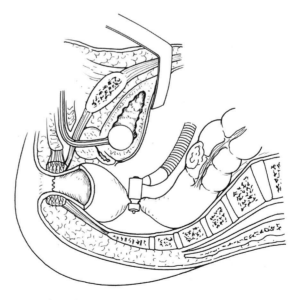

The instrument's head is designed to articulate completely on the shaft, which also rotates and flexes. In low anterior resections, this allows for a staple line perpendicular to the rectum.

Linear Cutters

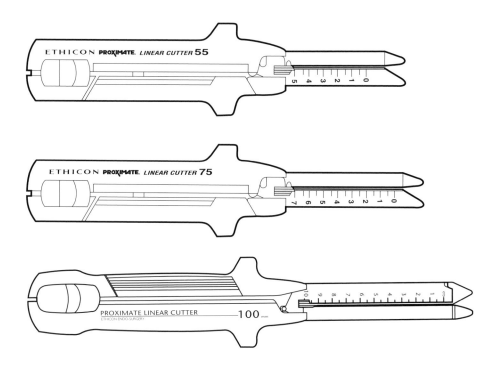

Linear cutters have applications in gastrointestinal, gynecologic, thoracic, and pediatric surgery to transect and resect tissues. They also can be used for the creation of certain types of anastomoses.

All three linear cutters have corresponding cartridges. The Compact Flex and 55-mm cutters are available with white, blue, and green cartridges and the 75-mm and 100-mm cutters are available in blue and green only. The cartridge color indicates the wire diameter and open and closed staple heights. Additionally, the 55-mm linear cutter is available without a knife (no-knife cutter). Every type of cartridge available in the same length is interchangeable on the same instrument.

A recent development was the shortening of the shaft of an endoscopic-type linear cutter for use in open procedures. This facilitates access and allows for one-handed versus the two-handed requirement of traditional linear cutters.

Do not use linear cutters on ischemic or necrotic tissue.

Linear cutters may be reloaded seven times during a single procedure.

Staple Lines

55-mm Linear Cutter

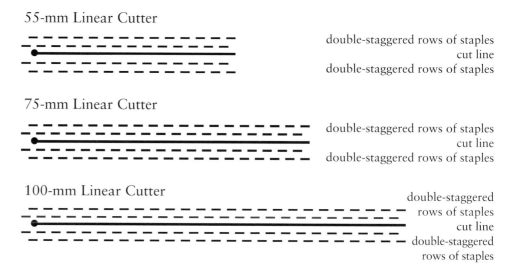

double-staggered rows of staples
cut line
double-staggered rows of staples

75-mm Linear Cutter

double-staggered rows of staples
cut line
double-staggered rows of staples

100-mm Linear Cutter

double-staggered
rows of staples
cut line
double-staggered
rows of staples

Linear cutters deliver two double-staggered rows of staples while simultaneously dividing the tissue between the rows.

The dot on the illustrations above indicates the end of the cut line.

The stapling and cutting mechanisms are synchronized, so that staple formation, which causes tissue adaptation and hemostasis in the wound area, is finished by compression before the tissue is actually cut and stapled.

The staple line is longer than the cut line to ensure hemostasis at the distal end of the staple line.

The process is shown in Figs. 1–4.

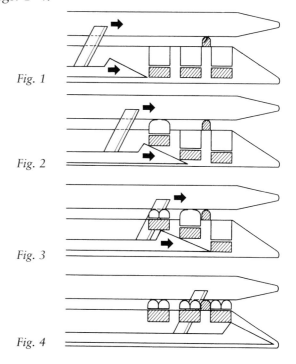

Fig. 1

Fig. 2

Fig. 3

Fig. 4

The tissue is stapled prior to knife activation (Fig. 1). The staple has been completely formed before the tissue is cut by the knife (Fig. 2–3). The cut line ends before the staple line (Fig. 4).

Circular Staplers

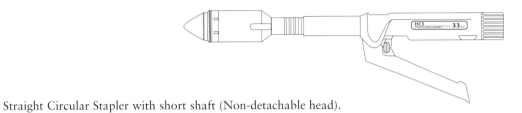

Straight Circular Stapler with short shaft (Non-detachable head).

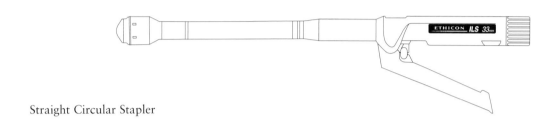

Straight Circular Stapler

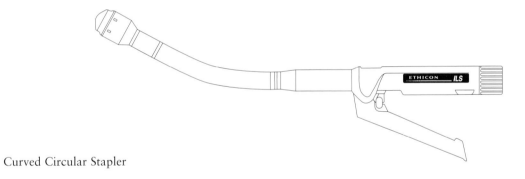

Curved Circular Stapler

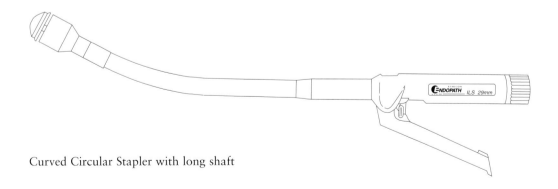

Curved Circular Stapler with long shaft

Circular staplers have applications in gastrointestinal surgery to facilitate inverted end-to-end, end-to-side, side-to-end, and side-to-side anastomoses. The straight circular stapler with short shaft (non-detachable head) is primarily indicated for the excision of prolapsed rectal mucosa.

The instruments, with the exception of the straight circular stapler with short shaft, are available in four different head diameters, which are selected depending on the lumen of the organ. Furthermore, the height of the staple closure can be varied intraoperatively from 1.0 mm to 2.5 mm, depending on the thickness of the structures to be anastomosed.

Because its shaft is sealed, the curved circular stapler with long shaft can also be used in minimally invasive surgical procedures.

Do not use circular staplers on ischemic or necrotic tissue. Furthermore, the instruments should not be used to create an anastomosis on structures where the combined tissue thickness is less than 1.0 mm or greater than 2.5 mm.

Circular staplers are not reloadable.

Circular staplers deliver a circular, double-staggerd row of staples, while simultaneously creating a uniform stoma between the organs to be anastomosed.

Staple Lines

21-mm Circular Stapler
Two staggered rows of staples
Variable staple height 1.0–2.5 mm

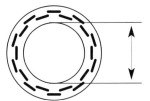

Internal lumen
Circular cut line
12.4-mm diameter

25-mm Circular Stapler
Two staggered rows of staples
Variable staple height 1.0–2.5 mm

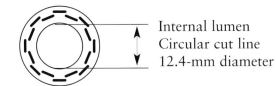

Internal lumen
Circular cut line
16.4-mm diameter

29-mm Circular Stapler
Two staggered rows of staples
Variable staple height 1.0–2.5 mm

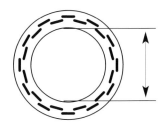

Internal lumen
Circular cut line
20.4-mm diameter

33-mm Circular Stapler
Two staggered rows of staples
Variable staple height 1.0–2.5 mm

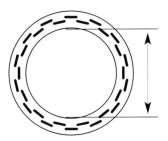

Internal lumen
Circular cut line
24.4-mm diameter

According to the principles of surgical stapling, the main objective is to create an anastomosis with the largest lumen possible in order to avoid stenosis.

Sizers

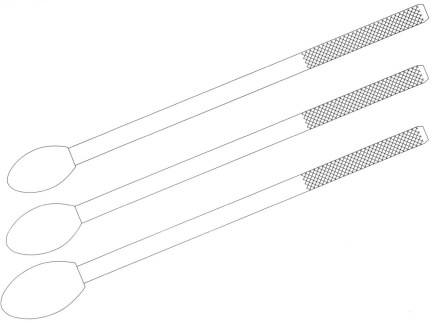

Circular sizers aid in selecting the appropriate circular stapler size. As previously mentioned, the objective is to create the largest lumen possible. After transecting the bowel, the lumen is dilated with the circular sizers. Care should be taken so that the bowel tissue layers do not tear.

The circular sizers are available in 25-mm, 29-mm, and 33-mm diameters, corresponding with the head sizes of the circular staplers. Begin sizing the bowel using the 25-mm circular sizer, and then continue with successively larger ones until the appropriate sizer fills the lumen.

Purse-String Suture Clamp

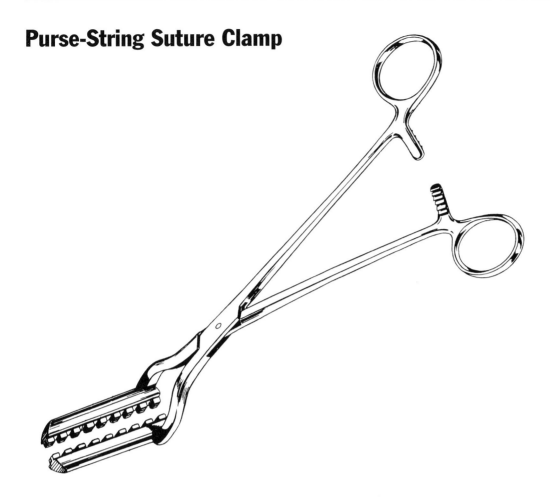

This instrument facilitates prompt placement of a purse-string suture.

After the clamp has been closed, adjustments will be possible only if the bowel segment damaged by the teeth of the clamp is resected. Ensure correct closure of the instrument prior to inserting needles into the canals.

Resection should be performed along the knife guide to achieve optimal distance between the purse-string suture and the cut tissue edge. The clamp must be removed carefully to avoid damaging the purse-string suture.

Be sure to inspect the purse-string suture.

For detailed information, refer to the chapter on purse-string suture techniques.

Do not use this instrument on ischemic or necrotic tissues.

Synthetic Absorbable Clips

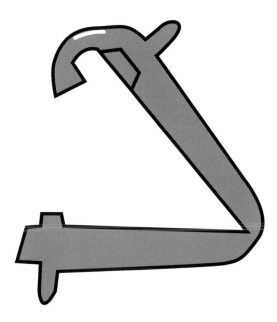

Synthetic absorbable ABSOLOK™ Clips are made of a polydioxanone polymer. During the absorption period, the clip causes minimal tissue reaction. The violet polydioxanone polymer reacts neither antigenically nor pyrogenically.

Breakdown occurs through hydrolysis, which produces H_2O and CO_2. These products are excreted by way of the urinary and respiratory systems. In the first 90 postoperative days, there is minimal absorption and also minimal loss of tensile strength. After 210 days the polydioxanone polymer is completely absorbed.

Synthetic absorbable clips are used for the ligation of vessels and tubular structures. The absorbable clips do not conduct heat or electricity. There is no interference with interpretations of radiological, CT, or MRI scans.

When using a ligating clip, it is important that the size of the clip be consistent with the tissue being ligated. Therefore, synthetic absorbable clips are available in four different sizes: small, medium, medium/large, and large.

Before a clip is used, the vessel to be ligated must be dissected to ensure proper placement of the clip around the structure. The ABSOLOK™ Clip has a self-locking mechanism that encircles the structure. After clip application, inspect the site for hemostasis and examine the locking mechanism for complete closure.

A wide range of clip appliers in different sizes and lengths is available for open and minimally invasive surgery.

Clip	Vessel Diameter (Ø)

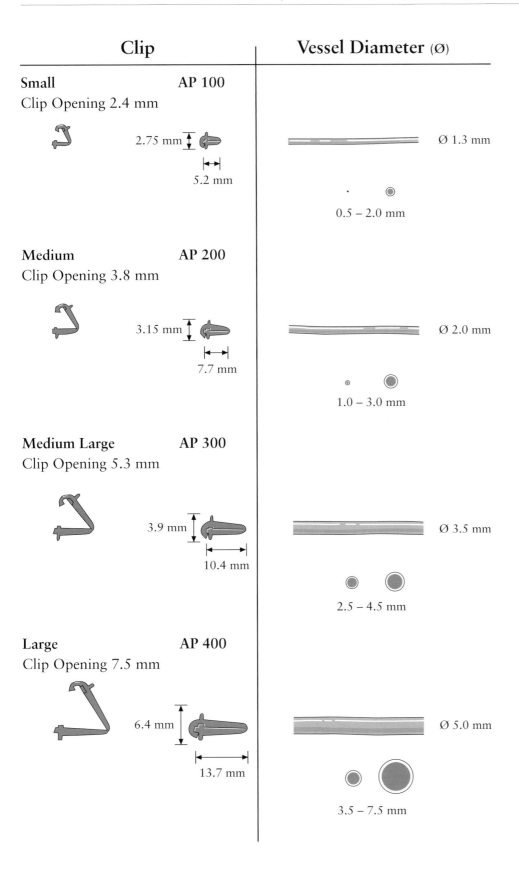

Small AP 100
Clip Opening 2.4 mm

2.75 mm
5.2 mm

Ø 1.3 mm

0.5 – 2.0 mm

Medium AP 200
Clip Opening 3.8 mm

3.15 mm
7.7 mm

Ø 2.0 mm

1.0 – 3.0 mm

Medium Large AP 300
Clip Opening 5.3 mm

3.9 mm
10.4 mm

Ø 3.5 mm

2.5 – 4.5 mm

Large AP 400
Clip Opening 7.5 mm

6.4 mm
13.7 mm

Ø 5.0 mm

3.5 – 7.5 mm

Metal Clips

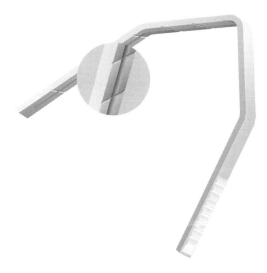

Non-absorbable ligating clips are used for the ligation of vessels and tubular structures. The ligating clips, particularly those made of titanium, can be used to mark internal structures, since they can be clearly identified on X-rays.

When using a ligating clip, it is important that the size of the clip be consistent with the tissue being ligated. Therefore, metal clips are available in four different sizes: small, medium, medium/large, and large.

The ligating clips are produced from either stainless steel or titanium. It is important to select the appropriate clip material prior to the procedure. Stainless steel clips may interfere with interpretations of postoperative X-rays, CT, or MRI scans, and therefore inhibit clear identification and assessment of surrounding structures.

Both stainless steel and titanium clips cause minimal tissue reaction.

Clip		Vessel Diameter (Ø)

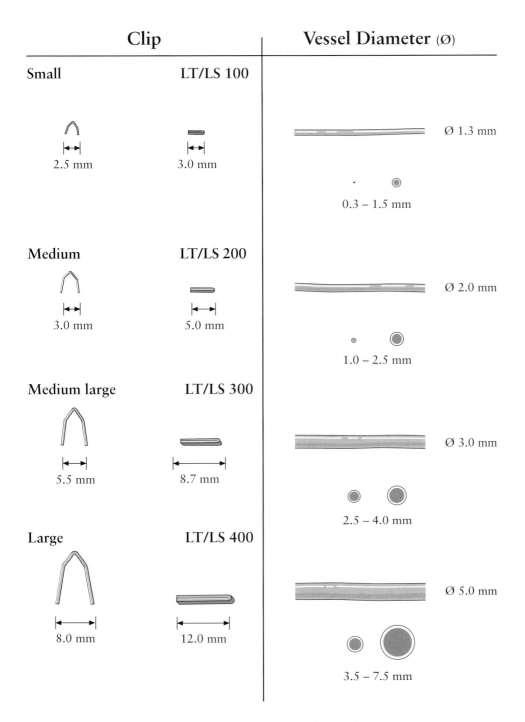

Small   **LT/LS 100**

2.5 mm   3.0 mm

Ø 1.3 mm

0.3 – 1.5 mm

Medium   **LT/LS 200**

3.0 mm   5.0 mm

Ø 2.0 mm

1.0 – 2.5 mm

Medium large   **LT/LS 300**

5.5 mm   8.7 mm

Ø 3.0 mm

2.5 – 4.0 mm

Large   **LT/LS 400**

8.0 mm   12.0 mm

Ø 5.0 mm

3.5 – 7.5 mm

To ensure clip security on the structure being ligated, lateral and transverse grooves are present on the innerside of the clip. This can be seen in the diagram on page 26. After clip application, inspect the site for hemostasis and ensure that each clip has been securely positioned around the structure being ligated. Metal clips conduct heat and electricity so special caution should be exercised when using electrosurgery.

A wide range of clip appliers in different sizes and lengths is available for open and minimally invasive surgery.

Multiple Clip Appliers

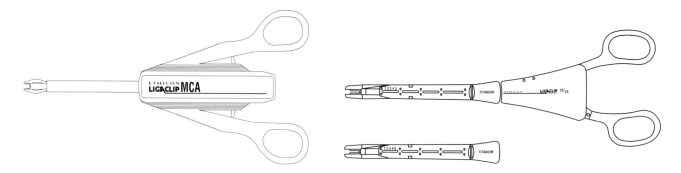

Multiple clip appliers are designed to provide quick, efficient ligation by means of an integrated mechanism that reloads the instrument automatically. Multiple clip appliers have a ratchet mechanism that prevents clips from being displaced from the jaws inadvertently.

Multiple clip appliers are available in different clip sizes and lengths, enabling comfortable use even at sites where access is difficult. For detailed information refer to the table below.

When using multiple clip appliers, adhere to the same principles as described with single clips.

Product Code	Applier Length	No. of Clips	Clip Size	Clip Open		Clip Distal Closure	Clip Closed	
MCS20	23.8 cm	20	small		2.1 mm			3.8 mm
MSM20	23.8 cm	20	medium		4.3 mm			6.0 mm
MCM20	29.2 cm	20	medium		4.3 mm			6.0 mm
MCM30	29.2 cm	30	medium		4.3 mm			6.0 mm
MCL20	33.7 cm	20	large		6.3 mm			10.8 mm
TIM20	29.4 cm	20	medium		4.4 mm			4.8 mm
TIR20 (Reload of TIM20)	–	20	medium		4.4 mm			4.8 mm

Skin Staplers

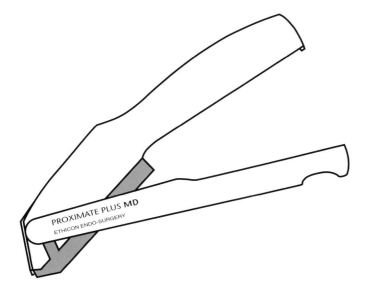

Skin staplers are designed for quick skin closure and good cosmetic results. When using skin staplers, ensure that the staples are at least 5 mm anterior to underlying structures such as bones, vessels, or other organs.

The instrument delivers staples one at a time. The distance between the applied staples should be approximately 8 mm. If the distance is more than 8 mm between the single staples, the cosmetic result may be unsatisfactory.

Evert wound edges during approximation.

A specially designed staple extractor should be used for staple removal.

unformed skin staple   formed skin staple

3 Basic Stapling Techniques

Over the years, various surgical stapling techniques have been developed and refined. The most common and basic uses of mechanical staplers for transections, ligations, and anastomoses of anatomical structures are described below.

Examples of the use of Linear Staplers:

Closure of Organs

Linear Staplers allow the closure of organs at a line of transection. The tissue to be stapled should be positioned into the open jaws of the linear stapler. Ensure that no clips or foreign bodies are included in the instrument's jaws. Intraluminal devices such as probes or catheters must be removed from the area to be stapled.

After the organ to be stapled is correctly positioned in the jaws, the instrument is closed and fired. Prior to opening the stapler, a clamp should be placed parallel to, and on the side of, the linear stapler's cutting guide to prevent any leakage from the opened end of the organ once it is transected. After the organ is transected along the stapler's cutting guide, open the instrument and inspect the wound edges for hemostasis.

In isolated cases, especially those involving heavily vascularized structures, staple line bleeding can be controlled with a suture ligature or the Harmonic Scalpel. When using electrosurgery to achieve hemostasis, any contact between staple and electrode must be avoided, since this may result in necrosis in the staple line area. The preferred method for attaining hemostasis is with a suture ligature or the Harmonic Scalpel. For more details on the Harmonic Scalpel, refer to Chapters 5 and 6.

When ligating small vessels or very thin tissue, the vascular stapler is used.

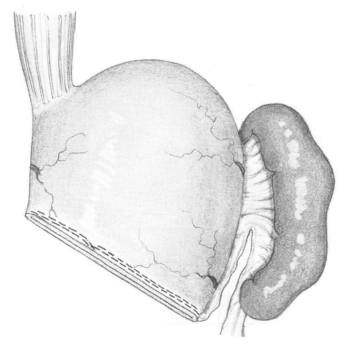

Closure of Otomies

When an anastomosis is created involving a hollow organ, hemostasis must be obtained prior to closing the otomy. As shown in the illustration, traction or stay sutures are used to elevate and help position the tissue into the instrument. This allows the tissue edges to be approximated before being stapled. After closing and firing the stapler, but prior to opening the instrument, the excess tissue protruding from the jaws is resected along the cutting guide using a scalpel or scissors.

When a linear stapler is used to perform a lateral closure of an otomy, care is taken to include as little tissue as possible in the instrument jaws to avoid stenosis. To minimize the risk of stenosis some surgeons choose to close a longitudinal otomy transversely.

After removing the linear stapler, examine the staple line for hemostasis. Isolated bleeding is controlled with suture ligatures or the Harmonic Scalpel.

In mechanical stapling, **a minimum distance of 3 cm** should be left between two staple lines to avoid risk of tissue necrosis due to vascular compromise in the tissue between the lines.

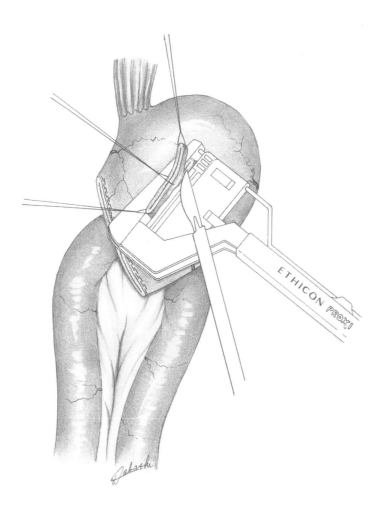

End-to-End Anastomosis: Triangulation Technique

An end-to-end anastomosis can be performed with the linear stapler. The instrument is fired three times to form the triangulation.

The mesenteric and antimesenteric borders of the two structures to be anastomosed must be properly aligned. Using traction or stay sutures, the three opposing sides are properly aligned to form the triangulation.

The posterior walls of the bowel segments to be anastomosed are inverted and stapled first. Resect any excess tissue protruding from the jaws of the instrument using the cutting guide. After creating the posterior wall anastomosis, the final two firings occur with the tissue edges in the everted position, ensuring that the two staple lines cross at their corners. This technique creates a large lumen, thereby decreasing the possibility of stenosis.

Once completed, the staple lines are examined for hemostasis. Isolated bleeding is controlled with suture ligatures or the Harmonic Scalpel.

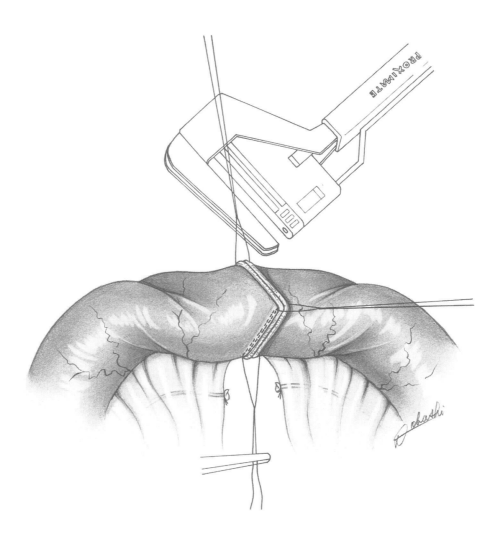

Examples of the use of Linear Cutters:

Transection of Tubular Structures and Organs

The linear cutter applies two double-staggered rows of staples and transection occurs between these rows. The tissue to be stapled should be evenly distributed between the forks of the instrument. The intermediate locking position on the linear cutter can be used while positioning the tissue.

Clips, probes, catheters, and similar foreign bodies must not be included in the instrument jaws. After transecting the tissue, examine the edges for hemostasis.

In isolated cases, especially those involving heavily vascularized structures, staple line bleeding can be controlled with a suture ligature When using electrosurgery to achieve hemostasis, any contact between staple and electrode must be avoided, since this may result in necrosis in the staple line area. The preferred method for attaining hemostasis is with a suture ligature or the Harmonic Scalpel.

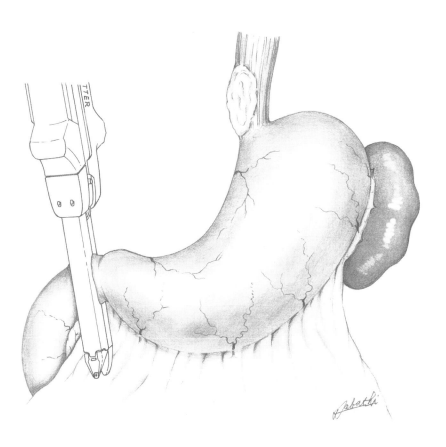

Creation of a Side-to-Side Anastomosis

The side-to-side anastomosis is created with the linear cutter. Using traction or stay sutures, approximate the bowel segments side by side, being certain to align the antimesenteric borders. Make a small opening into the lumen of both bowel segments on adjacent antimesenteric borders with a scalpel or the Harmonic Scalpel.

Insert one fork of the linear cutter into each bowel lumen. To facilitate the alignment of the tissue edges around the forks, the instrument can be placed in the intermediate locking position. The stapler is closed and fired.

The two segments are anastomosed with two double-staggered rows of staples. At the same time, the knife blade in the instrument divides the walls of the bowel between the two staple lines, creating a stoma.

The common opening is closed with a linear stapler or sutures. Before removing the stapler, use a scalpel or scissors along the cutting guide to excise any redundant tissue protuding through the jaws. A single safety stitch can be placed to avoid tension at the distal end of the new anastomosis.

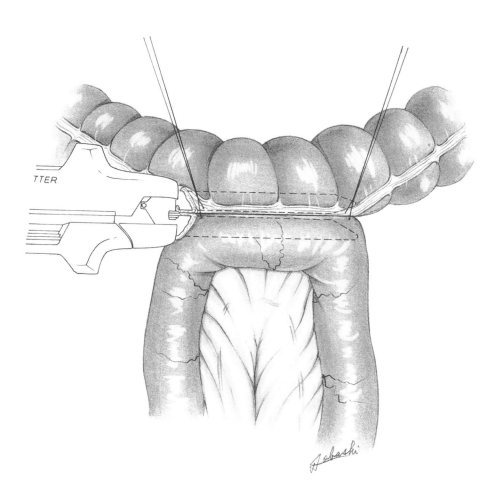

Creation of a Functional End-to-End Anastomosis – Closed Technique

The segment to be resected is mobilized using suture ligatures, clips, or the Harmonic Scalpel. Once mobilized, the proximal and distal lines of transection are created with the liner cutter. With this technique, both the patient and specimen ends of the bowel are stapled prior to transection, thereby reducing the possibility of intraperitoneal contamination.

The anastomosis is created with one firing of the linear cutter. The antimesenteric corners of the staple line closures of both segments are excised, and one fork of the linear cutter is inserted into each bowel lumen. To facilitate the alignment of the tissue edges around the forks, the instrument can be placed in the intermediate locking position. The stapler is closed and fired. Two double-staggered staple lines join the bowel walls and the knife blade in the instrument divides the walls between the two staple lines, creating a stoma.

The common opening is closed with a linear stapler or sutures. Before removing the stapler, use a scalpel or scissors along the cutting guide to excise any redundant tissue protuding through the jaws.

A single safety stitch can be placed to avoid tension at the distal end of the anastomosis.

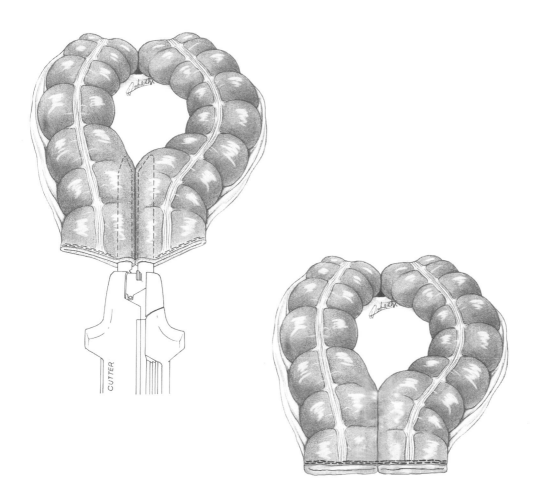

Pulmonary Wedge Resections with the Linear Cutter: Atypical/Non-Anatomic Resection

The specimen is excised with two overlapping firings of the linear cutter. By using the linear cutter, both tissue edges at the site of transection are stapled, thereby achieving hemostasis and pneumostasis.

After identifying the margins of the lesion, the linear cutter is positioned so the forks extend beyond the lesion. The instrument is closed and fired. To complete the resection, reapply the instrument so that the staple lines overlap at the apex of the wedge. The instrument is closed and fired, allowing the specimen to be removed. Examine the staple line for hemostasis and pneumostasis. Air leaks can be identified by filling the thoracic cavity with sterile saline solution and inflating the lung.

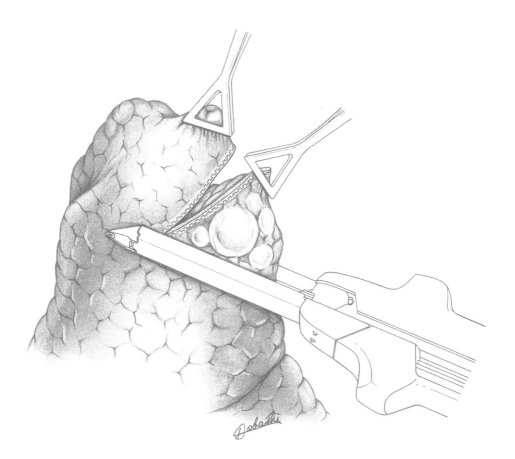

Examples of the use of Circular Staplers:

Circular staplers are primarily intended to create anastomoses between hollow and tubular organs. The end-to-end and end-to-side anastomoses are described below.

End-to-End Anastomosis via Colotomy with Circular Stapler

With this technique, the end-to-end anastomosis is created with one firing of the circular stapler through a colotomy. The colotomy is closed with a linear stapler.

The procedure begins with the mobilization of the diseased segment using suture ligatures, clips, or the Harmonic Scalpel. Once mobilized, the proximal and distal lines of transection are created with a linear cutter. The staple lines are then resected and purse-string sutures are placed at the proximal and distal margins of the resection (Non-crushing bowel clamps are placed proximally and distally to minimize spillage).

Using a scalpel or the Harmonic Scalpel, a colotomy is created on the antimesenteric side approximately 6–8 cm from one of the transected ends. The colotomy, which should be large enough to allow for the insertion of the circular stapler, may be created in either the proximal or distal segment of bowel.

An appropriately sized circular stapler is chosen. The anvil is detached and inserted into the lumen of the bowel segment without the colotomy. Stay sutures are used to facilitate the insertion of the anvil. Once the anvil is fully introduced into the bowel lumen, the purse-string suture is secured to the anvil shaft. The circular stapler is then inserted into the bowel lumen of the other segment through the colotomy. Open the instrument and position it so that the purse-string suture can be securely tied to the integral trocar.

After the two bowel segments have been properly aligned, the anvil is attached to the integral trocar, and the instrument is closed and fired. This creates an end-to-end anastomosis. As the instrument is fired, the staples are formed against the anvil. A circular knife blade advances to cut a uniform stoma between the proximal and distal segments.

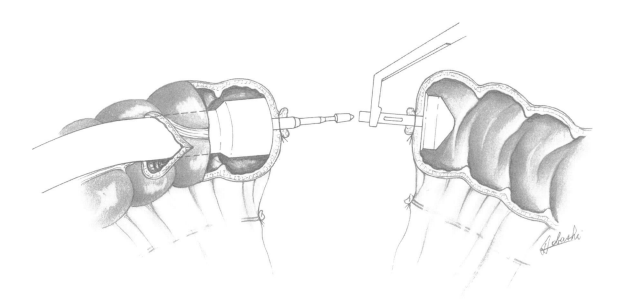

Before the stapler is withdrawn, the adjusting knob is turned counter clockwise $1/2 - 3/4$ turn. The instrument is gently rotated 90° to the right and then 180° to the left to ensure tissue release. The instrument is withdrawn and the tissue donuts are examined. The tissue donuts should be intact and include all tissue layers. If the donuts are not complete, the anastomosis should be carefully checked for leakage and appropriate repairs made.

The colotomy is closed with a linear stapler. Prior to removal of the stapler, the cutting guide is used to excise any redundant tissue protruding through the jaws.

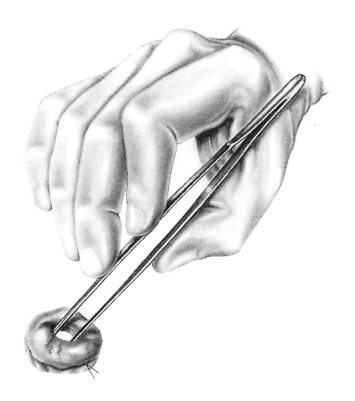

End-to-Side Anastomosis without Colotomy

Using this technique the anastomosis is created with a circular stapler and the intestine is closed with a linear stapler. The illustration below depicts a right hemicolectomy.

The procedure begins with the mobilization of the diseased segment, using suture ligatures, clips, or the Harmonic Scalpel. Once mobilized, the proximal and distal lines of transection are created with a linear cutter. The staple lines are then excised to expose the lumens of the terminal ileum and the distal bowel segment. (Instead of using the linear cutter, the proximal and distal lines of transection can be created between bowel clamps.) A purse-string suture is placed on the terminal ileum to accommodate the anvil of the circular stapler.

An appropriately sized circular stapler is chosen. The anvil is detached and inserted into the lumen of the terminal ileum. The purse-string suture is securely tied around the anvil center rod.

The circular stapler is inserted into the distal bowel lumen. The tip of the integral trocar is gently pressed against the antimesenteric aspect of the colon where the anastomosis will be created, perforating the bowel wall by fully extending the integral trocar.

After the bowel segments are properly aligned, the anvil is attached to the integral trocar. The circular stapler is closed and fired, creating the end-to-side anastomosis.

After the circular stapler is withdrawn the tissue donuts are examined for completeness. The donuts should be intact and include all tissue layers. If the donuts are not complete, the anastomosis should be carefully checked for leakage and appropriate repairs made.

The open segment of bowel is closed with a linear stapler. Prior to removing the stapler, use the cutting guide to excise any redundant tissue protruding through the jaws.

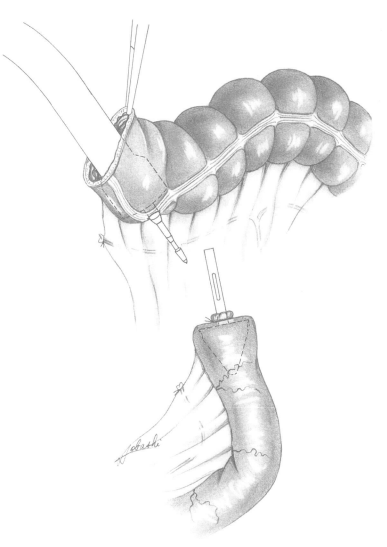

4 Purse-String Suture Techniques

In performing an anastomosis one of the critical factors for success is the proper placement of a purse-string suture. Clinical evidence has demonstrated that one of the main reasons anastomoses fail is an improperly placed purse-string suture, especially deep in the pelvis. Therefore, it is essential to have a good understanding of the principles involved in correctly placing a purse-string suture, and of the different techniques used.

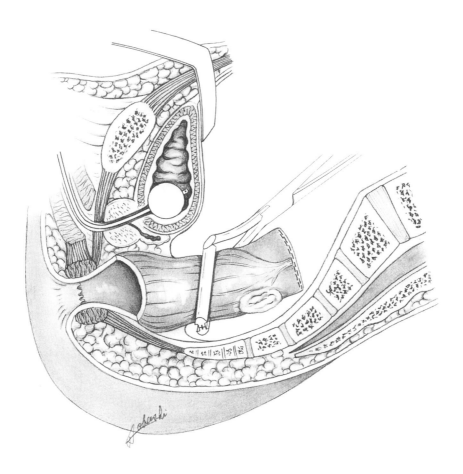

Principles of Placing a Purse-String Suture

A purse-string suture can be placed manually or with the aid of a purse-string suture clamp or device. In both approaches, a monofilament suture is chosen. A monofilament suture slides through the tissue easily and minimizes the risk of tissue trauma. To avoid damaging and weakening the suture, it should not be grasped with any instrument.

A manually placed purse-string suture should start at the antimesenteric border. This facilitates purse-string closure under direct visualization. The maximum distance of the needle stitches (which should include all tissue layers) should be 4 mm from the cut edge and 6 mm from puncture to puncture.

Hand-Sewn Purse-String Suturing Techniques

Standard "Through-and-Through"

The suturing includes all tissue layers and is performed by initially running the needle from external to internal to external and ending with the needle passing from internal to external. This technique has the advantage of easier pull-down while minimizing the tissue cuff and suture breakage.

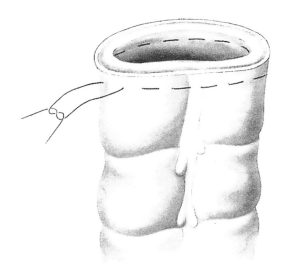

"Baseball" or Whip Stitch Purse-String Suturing

The suturing includes all tissue layers and is performed by always passing the needle from external to internal, including the tissue edges. The end of the suture is passed from internal to external. This technique is sometimes useful with a smaller diameter lumen.

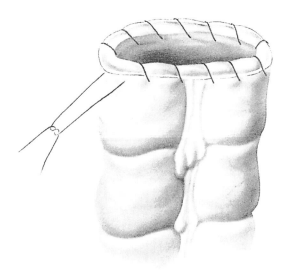

Whip Stitch with Loop

This technique is a variation of the previous one and is used in bowel with a large lumen. A long loop should be left after half of the circumference has been sutured to provide a second traction point during purse-string closure.

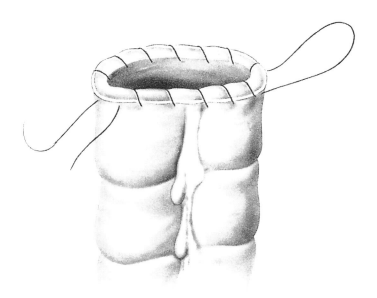

Whip Stitch with Two Sutures

This technique is a variation of the previous one, in that two separate sutures are used to create traction points.

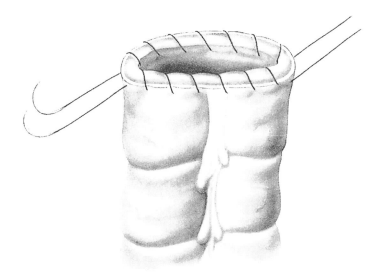

Thorlakson Clamp as an Aid

The Thorlakson clamp facilitates purse-string suturing by keeping the lumen of the bowel open.

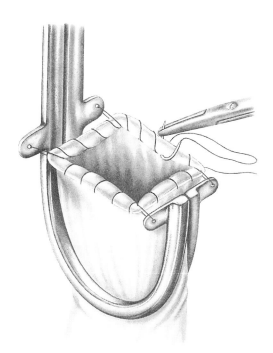

Techniques for Added Security in Creating a Purse-String

After the purse-string suture has been tied around the center rod of the stapler, additional security can be obtained by wrapping suture around it.

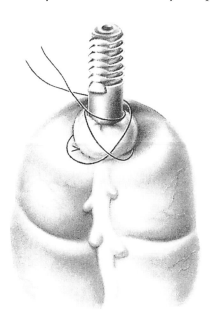

When the distance between the stitches is not uniform, an additional stitch needs to be placed in the gap to maintain the function of the purse-string.

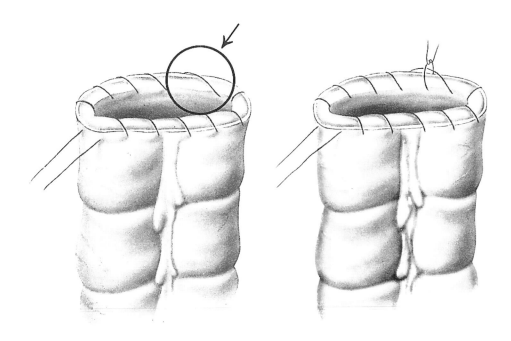

Purse-String Suture Clamp

In the area of the intended anastomosis the mesentery and fat are dissected away from the bowel wall to clear an area 1.5–2.0 cm in length. The clamp must be applied at a right angle, not obliquely. This prevents tissue from bunching up on one side in the circular stapler after the purse-string suture is tied. Following clamping, adjustments will only be possible if the bowel segment damaged by the teeth of the clamp is resected. If this is not done, postoperative complications due to ischemia and necrosis could occur.

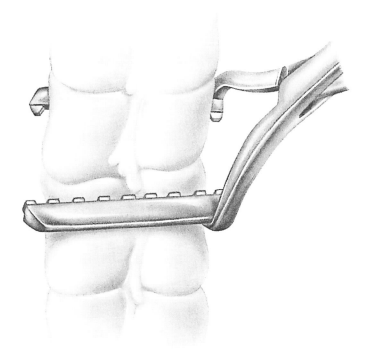

For placement of the purse-string suture, a 75-cm monofilament suture with two soft 60-mm ATRALOC™ straight needles is recommended. In narrow areas, the needle can be bent immediately after exiting the needle canal, so that it can be adjusted to the corresponding space.

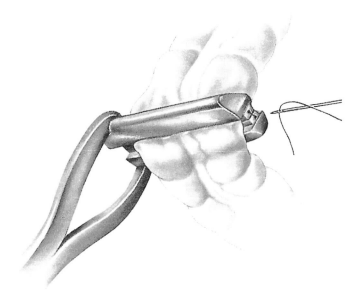

The bowel must be resected with a scalpel along the cutting edge of the purse-string suture clamp. This maintains an optimal distance between the purse-string suture and the cut tissue edge. There must be no excess tissue protruding beyond the purse-string suture. Any excess tissue would interfere with the proper functioning of the circular knife, and could result in the formation of incomplete tissue donuts. When the clamp is opened, ensure that the suture comes loose from the needle canals, and that the purse-string suture is complete.

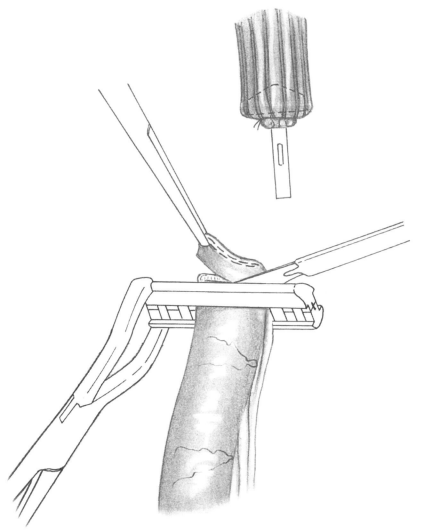

If desired, the purse-string suture clamp can be left in place for a prolonged period. There is no risk of necrosis because the tissue segment traumatized by the clamp is resected by the circular stapler.

5 UltraCision – The Harmonic Scalpel

In surgery, dissecting with minimal blood loss is of paramount importance. The range of possible indications is significantly influenced by the reliability of the technology employed for dividing tissues while securing hemostasis. Thick and/or adipose structures with numerous blood vessels (greater omentum, mesentery of the large and small intestine, regional lymph drainage areas) are particularly poorly accessible for video-endoscopic hemostasis. Safe video-endoscopic division of these anatomical structures usually exceeds the capacity of both high-frequency (HF) current techniques and video-endoscopic suturing.

Harmonic Scalpel technology was developed as an alternative method for achieving hemostasis. It was conceived primarily for minimally invasive surgery (MIS) in order to overcome the considerable disadvantages and risks associated with high-frequency technology. The rationale of the Harmonic Scalpel is the direct application of ultrasound for atraumatic surgical dissection and hemostasis that is gentle to the tissues.

Using Harmonic Scalpel technology, electrical energy is converted into mechanical energy by the generator in the handpiece, through a piezoelectric crystal system. The blade or tip of the instrument vibrates axially with a constant frequency of 55,500 Hertz. The longitudinal extension of the vibration can be varied between 25 and 100 μm in five levels. The energy liberated as an ultrasound wave is directly applied to the tissue.

The Harmonic Scalpel yields three possible effects: cavitation, coaptation/coagulation, and cutting. These effects can be applied to the tissue singly or in synergetic combination. The synergetic expression of these three effects depends on the type of tissue (water content), level selection on the generator (extension of longitudinal vibration), application time of energy, type and handling of the active instrument, and tension or pressure (or both) to the tissue.

Premises for the Development of the Harmonic Scalpel

In surgery, it is possible to divide small and larger blood vessels between ligatures during dissection or to control them by suturing them in the event of active bleeding. In addition, high frequency electrical coagulation (HF cautery) has been used in all branches of surgery for decades to deal with even the smallest sources of bleeding. HF cautery is used for cutting tissue as well as for hemostasis. The techniques of tissue division and hemostasis familiar from open surgery cannot be used in the usual way in video-endoscopic surgery. This circumstance has led to various compromise solutions and has hitherto appreciably narrowed the range of indications of MIS. The cautery "hook," used mainly for laparoscopic cholecystectomy, is suitable for dissection and division of anatomically distinct planes (non-infected cholecystectomy). The "hook," however, rapidly proves inadequate when local operating conditions are difficult, or when the range of indications of one's own video-endoscopic repertoire is being extended, especially regarding hemostasis. Classical surgical dissection technique (forceps, scissors) can be used in MIS until bleeding or preliminary hemostasis requires clamps to be applied and ligatures or transfixation placed under "open" conditions. A comparable situation can occur in MIS, but is then more difficult to resolve. Even for an expert surgeon, placing clips, suture loops, or transfixion sutures, or the use of stapling devices, is often tedious, time-consuming, cost-intensive, and surgically unsatisfactory.

The limited technical possibilities previously prevented extension of the range of indications of video-endoscopic surgery. On the other hand, they have stimulated the development of new technology, such as the Harmonic Scalpel.

The Harmonic Scalpel may replace high-frequency electrosurgery, which is associated with many disadvantages and risks, both in open and minimally invasive surgery.

The concept of ultrasound dissection was first developed for videoscopic surgery. General acceptance of this new technology very rapidly favored the practical use of the Harmonic Scalpel in all fields of surgical activity, thus launching a variety of new instruments.

Electrosurgery

Electrosurgery is routinely used to cut and coagulate body tissue with high-frequency (HF) electrical current, also known as radio-frequency (RF) current. Proper care and handling of electrosurgical equipment is essential to patient and personnel safety.

Current Density

An electrosurgical generator (ESU) supplies RF current to the active electrode. Current passes from the active electrode, through the patient, exits through the return electrode, and returns to the generator to complete the circuit. Without this complete circular path, from generator to patient and back again, current will not flow.

Current density is one of the most important concepts in electrosurgery. Simply stated, current density represents the amount of current per unit area. When a constant amount of current is produced by an ESU, the amount of the thermal effect produced at a given contact point will be inversely related to the size (area) of the contact point.

Monopolar vs. Bipolar Electrosurgery

In monopolar electrosurgery, the tissue effect takes place at the active electrode only. The dispersive electrode provides the path of least resistance from the patient back to the generator. No electrosurgical effect is intended or desired at the site of the dispersive electrode.

Bipolar electrosurgery provides a more delicate alternative. In bipolar electrosurgery, the active electrode is comprised of two individual tines. Current flows from the tip of one tine, through the tissue, to the tip of the other tine. Therefore, no dispersive pad is required. Limiting the flow of current to the small area between these two tiny contact points affords the surgeon greater control over the electrode's cutting or coagulating effects. Lateral thermal damage to sensitive nerves and vessels in close proximity to the instrument can be minimized. There is less chance of capacitive or direct arcing of current to surrounding structures, such as the bowel, and patient burns are virtually eliminated.

Ground-Referenced vs. Isolated Power Systems

Ground-referenced ESUs deliver electrical energy from the generator to the patient and back to the generator, which is connected to ground. Since an electrical current seeks to return to ground through the path of least resistance, it can flow through any grounded alternative path, such as an ECG pad. An isolated power system utilizes a large transformer assembly that converts conventional AC ground-referenced power to isolated power that has no voltage reference to ground. This is an important safety feature, because it reduces the risk of alternate-path burns.

Discrete vs. Nondiscrete Output

With discrete output, several active instruments may be attached to the ESU, but only one accessory may be activated at a time. The current will flow only through one accessory on a "first-come, first-served" basis. This is a safety factor of major importance to the surgical staff. With non-discrete output, when one accessory is activated, any and all accessories connected to the unit are also activated. All additional accessories must be isolated from the operative site.

Some manufacturers have developed "discrete output, simultaneous on-demand" capabilities. These units are still discrete; however, power may be shared between the two active electrodes. Thus, two surgeons may activate accessories simultaneously in the same mode. Because current follows the path of least resistance, it will split unevenly between the active electrodes. The majority of the AC current will flow to the tissue that offers the least impedance, and less current will flow to the higher impedance tissue. When one surgeon ceases activation, the other surgeon once again receives full power.

Electrosurgical Tissue Effects

Cutting

The first clinical mode of a modern ESU is cutting – either a pure cut or a blended cut. Pure cut is generally used for dissection. A blended cut adds some hemostatic effect. In the pure cut mode, the active electrode performs much like a stainless-steel scalpel; it provides little or no control over bleeding.

A surgeon experienced in electrosurgery knows how much current to use for a given type of tissue, procedure, and electrode size and shape. Thus, the amount of current to use is a personal clinical judgment, acquired primarily by experience.

When cutting with steel, speed is not a factor. With a pure cut current, the speed with which the surgeon makes the cut affects the width and depth of the cut. If the surgeon moves the active electrode fast enough, most of the heat energy generated by the electrode will stay in the thin layer of tissue next to the electrode. Faster cuts are fine and thin with minimal lateral tissue necrosis. Slower cutting destroys more cells, extending the area of destruction on either side of the cut and resulting in a deeper, wider incision.

While a stainless steel scalpel requires some pressure to make an incision, electrosurgical cutting is virtually effortless. With only a light, deft stroke, the electrode makes sharply defined incisions with relative ease. If the power is correctly adjusted, the active electrode should encounter little physical resistance. At the leading edge, current density is so high that a thin layer of cells directly in its path is literally vaporized, leaving behind a well defined incision. This means that the surgeon must carefully control the depth to which the electrode penetrates and must actively guide its path of travel in all dimensions.

A blended cut mode modulates the current waveform and adds off-time to the duty cycle, resulting in a blend of surgical effects. The blended cut allows the surgeon to cut and coagulate at the same time. In a pure cut mode, heat energy is so great that cells vaporize. With a blended cut, cell wall explosion and vaporization are replaced by the slow dehydration of cellular fluid and protein. This stops the bleeding at the moment the cut is actually being made. By adjusting the blend, the surgeon can get varying degrees of hemostasis.

"Intelligent" electrosurgical systems use a different method of providing hemostasis in the cutting modality. Instead of modulating the current waveform and adding off-time to the duty cycle, as in a blended cut, these microprocessor-controlled units sense total impedance at the site of the active electrode and automatically adjust the voltage, current, or power to optimize clinical performance. By not modulating the waveform and keeping peak voltage relatively low, there is no carbonization of the tissue, and coagulum buildup on the cutting electrode is greatly reduced. Voltage-controlled "intelligent" electrosurgical systems allow the surgeon to achieve a clinically reproducible cutting effect, independent of tissue resistance, electrode size, or speed of cut.

Coagulation

The ability to coagulate is one of the greatest advantages electrosurgery offers over a scalpel. Rather than just cutting, the surgeon can also make use of the desiccating effects of heat energy to seal off bleeding vessels. RF current can easily generate enough heat in living tissue to vaporize cells instantly if the current at the electrode is fairly constant. Interruptions in the flow of current give the tissues time to cool; therefore, instead of cells exploding, the slow drying out of the tissues causes coagulation. Heat is still generated in the tissue, but it is not sufficient to explode the cell membrane. Rather, the reduced heat energy dehydrates the protein and fluid content of cells.

With pinpoint coagulation an interrupted current causes controlled dehydration as the surgeon holds the electrode in physical contact with or against the tissue. The drying-out effects of a pure coagulating current produce a zone of coagulation necrosis that is limited to the surface layers of the tissue. Factors affecting pinpoint coagulation include current density, period of contact, and surgical technique. The tip should make only light, momentary contact with the surface, but the contact may be repeated if necessary. Power should be adequate to stop the bleeding.

Fulguration is another type of coagulation, in which the surgeon holds the electrode some distance away from the tissue. The RF current is delivered to tissue when sparks "jump" from the active electrode, across the air space, and come in contact with the tissue. The effect is greater depth of penetration and more rapid dehydration. Many factors can affect fulguration. Because the sparks must jump an air gap, the temperature and humidity of the surrounding air can change the results. The proximity of the electrode to the tissue will also affect the clinical results. Good fulguration technique helps avoid charring. The secret is to keep the electrode moving at all times to prevent the buildup of heat in one area. Usually, the surgeon moves the electrode over the area to be treated until a thick, leathery mass called an eschar forms on the tissue surface. The ideal effect is coagulation without a blackened eschar.

The Dispersive Electrode

Patient/pad contact is of utmost importance in preventing pad-related burns. Even a small loss of contact can increase current density, resulting in a burn, especially when using high power settings. There are several factors that influence the amount of contact between the pad and the patient, including pad stiffness, edge construction, and pad size.

Most modern ESUs are capable of monitoring pad contact. This is a very important feature for preventing pad-related burns. It's easy to identify a sensing pad, as it has two foil contacts.

Although some systems do a much more accurate job of monitoring than other systems, most work the same way. A small current is sent up one side of the pad, across the patient's skin, and returned through the other side of the pad. If part of the pad is removed from the patient's skin, the generator senses the change in resistance and an alarm sounds. More advanced systems also take into consideration the amount of power being used during the surgical procedure and allow more of the pad to be removed if lower power settings are being used. This prevents unnecessary alarms and interruptions.

Cavitation, Coaptation and Coagulation, Cutting

The new Harmonic Scalpel technology avoids all of the disadvantages of conventional HF surgery. Application of ultrasound to the tissues allows three effects to act synergetically at all times: cavitation, coaptation/coagulation, and cutting.

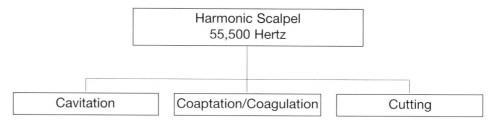

Cavitation

Cavitation describes the formation and disappearance of vapor bubbles in flowing liquids when the velocity is altered (Fig. 1). If the pressure falls below the vapor pressure of the liquid under acceleration in a flowing liquid, vapor mist forms in the liquid. With subsequent slowing, the pressure rises again, causing condensation. The large alterations of volume give rise to vigorous surges of pressure, which lead to sound radiation and damage to solid bodies. This phenomenon occurs, for example, in turbines, valves, and propellers.

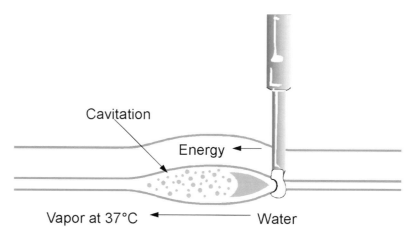

Fig. 1 Cavitation by application of ultrasound to the tissue causes dissection of tissue planes by water vaporization at body temperature.

With the Harmonic Scalpel, cavitation occurs the other way round – by means of high-frequency vibration of a solid body. The vibration is transmitted to the tissues, and this causes rapid volume changes in the tissue and cell fluid. This in turn leads to the formation of vapor bubbles at body temperature. In the parenchyma, cells explode. In connective tissue, bubble formation leads to the dissection of tissue planes.

Use of cavitation to dissect tissue planes is especially beneficial in anatomically inaccessible regions or in the vicinity of vulnerable structures. In exposing the esophagus in preparation for laparoscopic fundoplication, for example, the Harmonic Scalpel shears allow the surgeon to work with unobstructed vision and without bleeding.

Coaptation and Coagulation

Coaptation (Latin *coaptare* fasten, fit) means the adherence or welding together of tissues. When ultrasound and pressure are used on tissue simultaneously, the tertiary hydrogen bonds in proteins are disrupted. This fragmentation of protein compounds leads to the adherence of collagen molecules at low temperatures (from body temperature to a maximum of 63°C). When the locally applied energy acts for longer periods, there is also a rise in temperature, leading to the thermally induced release of water vapor (63°C to 100°C) and later to coagulation (denaturing of protein) at a maximum temperature of 150°C.

Coaptation is used for preliminary hemostasis in laparoscopic cholecystectomy. Application of ultrasound energy to the tissue and simultaneous exertion of pressure leads to sealing of superficial vessels, which can then be divided without bleeding.

In coagulation, the ultrasound energy is applied to the tissue, together with pressure, for longer periods (a few seconds). The additional thermal effect causes coagulation (denaturing) of proteins as well as coaptation (fragmentation).

Cutting

By using tension, pressure, or both, the tissue is rapidly stretched beyond its elastic limit by the high-frequency vibration and is cut smoothly by a sharp blade or instrument tip. In cholecystectomy, for instance, a dissecting blade is used which is similar to the cautery hook familiar from HF surgery.

The effect of cutting can be explained by the "rubber band phenomenon": if a scalpel blade is applied to an unstretched rubber band, the band will retreat because of its elasticity. However, if the rubber band is stretched, a light touch of the blade suffices to cut through it.

Local Tissue Temperature

When the Harmonic Scalpel is used, in contrast to HF cautery, no electric current is sent through the patient. All the risks associated with the direct use of electric current are thus avoided.

The various effects of the Harmonic Scalpel in tissues are achieved at temperatures up to a maximum of 150°C. Coaptation leads to fragmentation of proteins, and coagulation to denaturing of protein compounds (Fig. 2).

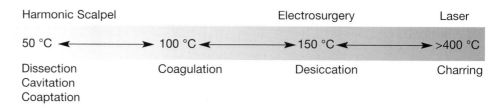

Fig. 2 Local tissue temperature with The Harmonic Scalpel, electrosurgery and laser.

Cavitation occurs at body temperature, coaptation in the range between body temperature and below 100°C, and coagulation at a temperature of up to 150°C. In this way there is no burning, carbonization, or smoke formation, as is the case with cautery or laser when temperatures of up to 400°C are reached (Fig. 3).

Temp. (°C)	Visual Change	Biological Change
37 - 50	Swelling	Heating, Retraction, Reduced Enzyme Activity
50 - 65	Blanching	Coagulation
65 - 90	White/Gray	Protein Denaturation
90 - 100	Puckering	Drying of Tissue
> 100	Drying	H_2O Boils, Cell Explosion
> 150	Charring	Carbonization
300 - 400	Blackening	Smoke Generation

Fig. 3 Macroscopic and microscopic tissue changes with the Harmonic Scalpel, electrosurgery, and laser at various local tissue temperatures.

Depth of Energy Penetration

When HF cautery is used, the maximum depth of penetration (Fig. 4) of the thermal electrical effect is reached soon after application of the HF current. With the Harmonic Scalpel, however, the depth of penetration of the energy flow (measured in mm) is correlated linearly with time (measured in seconds). The possibility of deeper penetration of tissue can be controlled more precisely with the Harmonic Scalpel using the "application time" factor.

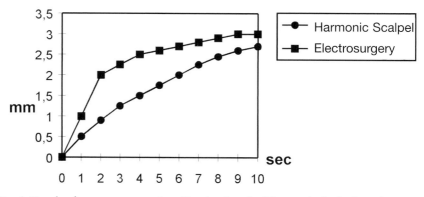

Fig. 4 Depth of energy penetration (liver) using the Harmonic Scalpel or electrocautery.

After an application time of about 5 seconds, which may not be exceeded during practical use of the Harmonic Scalpel, the depth of penetration is less than half of that in HF cautery. In practice, this is demonstrated by the fact that coagulation using the Harmonic Scalpel to achieve an effect equivalent to HF cautery always takes longer, but the effect on tissues is more readily controllable.

Apart from the depth of penetration of the energy, the temperature in the tissues and therefore the risk of unwanted thermal injury is considerably lower.

Lateral Energy Spread

Lateral spread of the energy flow and the effect that can be achieved with it reaches submaximum values after 3 seconds when HF cautery is used (Fig. 5). With the Harmonic Scalpel, there is a linear correlation between the time of application and the lateral spread of the effective energy flow.

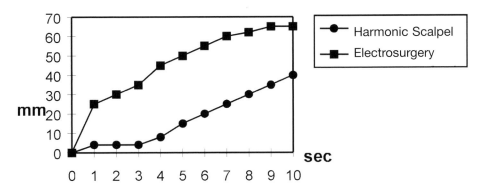

Fig. 5 Lateral spread of energy (liver) using the Harmonic Scalpel or electrocautery.

The risk of distant tissue damage is lower than in HF cautery, because of the lower lateral spread of the coagulation zone per se, and because the effect is controllable through the time factor.

Safe use of the Harmonic Scalpel allows low-risk dissection even close to vulnerable structures (e.g., bowel, ureter, blood vessels) where the use of HF cautery is ruled out or carries a high potential for risk.

Technological advantages of the Harmonic Scalpel

- No electrical current flow through the patient
- No risk of burns to the patient
- No distant tissue damage due to unnoticed current leakages
- Minimal carbonization of tissue
- Minimal smoke formation
- Minimal depth effect, minimal lateral propagation of the energy flow
- No neuromuscular stimulation
- No neutral electrode
- No risk of electric shocks or burns for the surgeon

Synergy – The Principle of Practical Use

The possible effects of the Harmonic Scalpel – cavitation, coaptation/coagulation, and cutting – can always be used as single functions or in any chosen modified synergetic combination (Fig. 6).

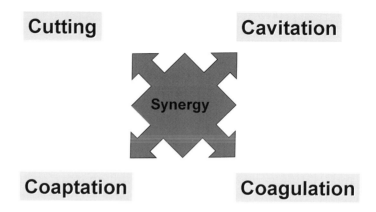

Fig. 6 Synergy of four Harmonic Scalpel qualities: Cavitation, Cutting, Coaptation, Coagulation

The effect of the applied ultrasound energy on tissue depends on the following parameters:

• Type of tissue (parenchyma, connective tissue)
• Water content of the tissue
• Setting of the device (variation of amplitude at 5 levels)
• Type of instrument blade used
• Exertion of tension, pressure, or both on the tissue
• Duration of energy effect on the tissue

The amplitude of the axial vibration of the tip of the instrument can be set on the generator at 5 levels. At level 1 the axial amplitude of vibration (deflection of tip of instrument in its longitudinal axis) is 25 µm. The frequency of the ultrasound energy (55,500 Hertz) is not affected by this setting. At level 5 the amplitude of the vibration of the tip of the instrument is 100 µm. The vibration frequency is 55,500 Hertz. Each instrument type (sharp, blunt, pointed, flat) has its own characteristics.

The desired effect of ultrasound energy on the tissue depends on the synergistically combined application of ultrasound energy and mechanical force (tension and/or pressure on the tissue). When shears are used, the side of the instrument blade selected (sharp, blunt, flat) is pressed against the Teflon-coated tissue pad with a variable degree of force (Fig. 7). In addition, variable tension on the tissue can be exerted overall with the closed instrument. The "strength" of the ultrasound energy is selected by choosing the amplitude of the axial vibration of the blade (level 1–5), and the amount of applied ultrasound energy is determined by the "application time" factor.

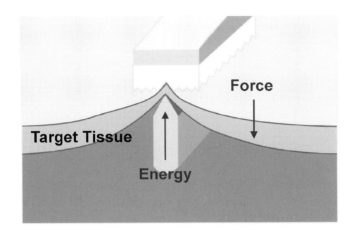

Fig. 7 Shears: the direction of energy is parallel to the applied force.

Cavitation is associated with the presence of water and is therefore employed predominantly in tissues with a high water content (Fig. 8). On the other hand, cutting is preferred in tissues with an extremely low water content (e.g., fascia).

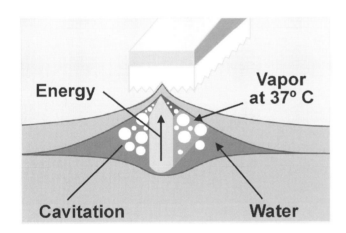

Fig. 8 Low pressure at the blade tip causes fluid to vaporize at low temperature. Cavitation causes separation of tissue planes.

Sharp blades, exertion of tension or pressure (or both) on the tissues, and high amplitude (level 5) lead to rapid tissue dissection/transection. Blunt blades or instrument tips, low tension or pressure in the tissues, and low amplitude (level 1–3) lead to coaptation and coagulation, depending on the time of effect of the energy.

Practical Use

The practical use of the Harmonic Scalpel entails a considerable change in technique for the surgeon who is used to high-frequency electrosurgery. A basic requirement for a successful changeover is precise knowledge and understanding of the technical basis and characteristics of the Harmonic Scalpel, and the necessary patience. Experience has shown that there are periods in the course of implementation of the Harmonic Scalpel:

The learning phase is limited to the first two weeks. During this time, the basic functions of the Harmonic Scalpel are experienced, step by step, in practical use, and can be converted for one's own applications.

> *Attending appropriate theoretical and practical courses can shorten the learning phase*

Although the Harmonic Scalpel was developed primarily for use in laparoscopic surgery, it seems reasonable during the initial learning phase to first try out the Harmonic Scalpel in selected open-surgery cases. Attempting to use the Harmonic Scalpel blades as cauterizers first results in mainly negative experiences. Putting into practice theoretical knowledge of the significance of tension and pressure, and of the need for a counterpressure for hemostasis, leads rapidly to acceptance and understanding of the functions of the Harmonic Scalpel.

After the first practical experiences in open surgery, use of the dissecting blades for laparoscopic surgery presents few or no problems. Lysis of adhesions and cholecystectomy are recommended as suitable initial operations. The absence of the otherwise very intrusive smoke and the possibility of risk-free dissection close to hilar structures in comparison to cautery, rapidly make themselves obvious as particular advantages in laparoscopic cholecystectomy.

> *In a habituation phase of a further two to four weeks, the surgeon builds knowledge of basic functions and applications, then employs the Harmonic Scalpel for general use in his or her personal operating repertoire.*

After the habituation period, the surgeon will have adapted the advantages of the new technology to his/her individual surgical technique. In the utilization phase, the Harmonic Scalpel can be used in all open and minimally invasive (elective and acute) operations. HF cautery can be replaced completely by the Harmonic Scalpel; thus, attachment of a neutral electrode (for safety) can be omitted.

6 The Harmonic Scalpel – System Components

The Harmonic Scalpel system components consist of the generator and transport cart, the footswitch, the handpiece, and the instruments that are connected to it (Fig. 9).

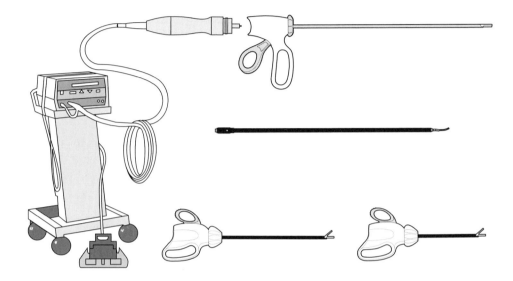

Fig. 9 The Harmonic Scalpel: System components, shears, and blades to be connected to the handpiece.

Generator, Footswitch, and Handpiece

The generator is connected to a regular power supply. The footswitch, which activates the output of the generator, has two pedals. The left pedal selects ultrasound energy from five levels (25–100 µm of longitudinal extension of vibration). On the right pedal the level is fixed at 5 (100 µm).

The handpiece contains the ultrasonic transducer and the ultrasonic amplifier (Fig. 10). The generator provides the electrical energy to be converted to ultrasonic energy at the piezoelectric ceramic pieces in the handpiece. The generator also allows continuous monitoring of the ultrasonic function. Irregularities of ultrasonic vibrations in any part of the system result in a continuous acoustic signal and the immediate shutdown of the system.

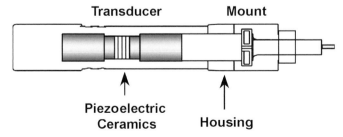

Fig. 10 Handpiece with ultrasonic transducer. Electrical energy is converted into ultrasonic vibration in a piezoelectric ceramic system. Energy is transferred to the blade systems by an acoustic mount coupled to the housing of the handpiece.

Instruments

The Harmonic Scalpel offers a wide range of blades and shears which, when connected to the handpiece, allow surgeons to perform cutting, coagulation, dissection, and grasping of tissue in both open, conventional surgery and minimally invasive surgery. All of the blades and shears are securely attached to the handpiece with a torque wrench.

Harmonic Scalpel Blades

Blades come in two types according to diameter: 10 mm and 5 mm

The 10-mm blades come in two different lengths, depending on whether they are to be used in conventional surgery (short blades: 10 cm), or in minimally invasive surgery (long blades: 30 cm).

The long 10-mm blades have three different tips according to the desired surgical application (Fig. 11):

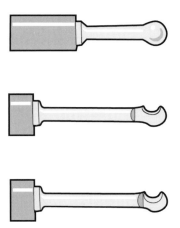

Fig. 11 10-mm instruments. The blade tips are configured as ball coagulator, blunt dissecting hook, and sharp hook.

- *Dissecting hook:* pointed, curved (60° radius of curvature) blade with a blunt outer edge, a sharp inner edge, and a sharp tip.
- *Sharp hook:* pointed, curved (40° radius of curvature) blade with a blunt outer edge, an even sharper inner edge, and a sharp tip.
- *Ball coagulator:* spherical-tip blade.

The blunt outer edge in both the dissecting and sharp hooks is used especially for cavitation, point hemostasis, and, to a certain extent, cutting. It corresponds in handling to a poker-like dissecting hook used in HF electrosurgery, and is therefore recommended as a primary instrument during training.

The pointed, sharp, curved blade, on the other hand, is specially designed for cutting. It is more precise in the application of ultrasonic energy. With these sharp edges less tension and pressure are needed for cutting. However, the possibility of bleeding while using the sharp edge, if coaptation has not been adequate, is higher than when using the blunt edge.

The flat side of the blade on both the sharp and dissecting hooks can be used for hemostasis, as can the blunt outer edge. It should be borne in mind that pressure must be exerted on the tissue, in contrast to HF cautery.

The ball coagulator is used to coagulate broad and diffuse areas of bleeding, e.g., bleeding from the liver bed after cholecystectomy.

The short 10-mm blade has only one tip configuration, corresponding to that of the sharp hook (Fig. 12).

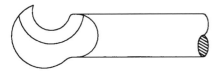

Fig. 12 Design of the 10-mm short blade: blunt outer edge, sharp inner edge, sharp tip.

The 5-mm blades come in three different lengths.

The short 5-mm blades, to be used in open/conventional surgery, have two lengths: 10 and 14 cm, depending on the surgeon's preference and the procedures to be performed.

The short 5-mm blades have three tip configurations:

- **Dissecting hook:** pointed, curved (60° radius of curvature) blade with a blunt outer edge, a sharp inner edge, and a sharp tip.
- **Sharp hook:** pointed, curved (40° radius of curvature) blade with a blunt outer edge, an even sharper inner edge, and a sharp tip.
- **Curved tip:** sharp edges on both sides to permit easy cutting in both directions. The concave and convex sides of the blade allow for coagulation, cavitation, and coaptation of tissue. The blunt tip will also facilitate spot coagulation for bleeding points. Because of the blade's curvature, the surgeon will have better visibility and easier access to areas otherwise difficult to reach (Figs. 13–15).

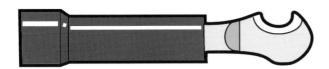

Fig. 13 5-mm sharp blade.

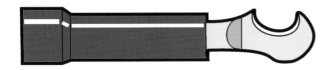

Fig. 14 5-mm dissecting blade.

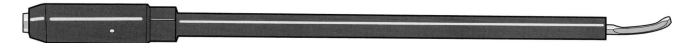

Fig. 15 5-mm curved blade.

The **long 5-mm blades** (32 cm) have applications in minimally invasive surgery. They come in four tip configurations:

- **Dissecting hook:** same as the short 5-mm blade.
- **Sharp hook:** same as the short 5-mm blade.
- **Curved tip:** same as the short 5-mm blade.
- **Ball coagulator:** spherical-tip blade.

Laparosonic Coagulating Shears

There are two type of shears also based on diameter: 10 mm and 5 mm.

The **10-mm shears** come in two lengths:

Short (20 cm), for open/conventional surgery.

Long (34 cm), for minimally invasive surgery.

Both shears consist of a grip housing and a multifunctional blade inside it. In addition, both shears have two types of handgrip configuration: pistol grip and scissor grip (Fig. 16).

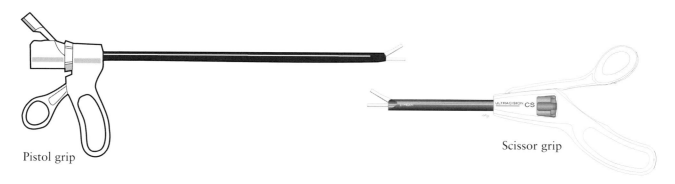

Pistol grip

Scissor grip

Fig.16 Laparosonic Coagulating Shears with pistol and scissor grip.

The tip of the shears has a mobile non-active branch (Teflon coated) that allows grasping and blunt dissection of tissue as well as its compression toward the ultrasonic non-mobile active blade.

The multifunctional active blade has three sides (sharp, blunt, and flat) that can be adjusted against the tissue pad (Fig. 17).

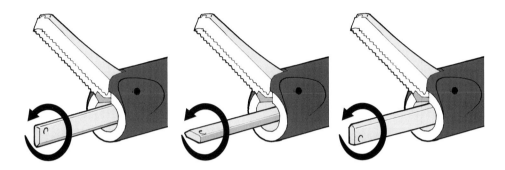

Fig. 17 The Laparosonic Coagulating Shears have three modes of blade configuration: blunt, flat, and sharp side.

The sharp edge is designed for cutting tissue. Hemostasis occurs only to a very limited extent with this setting, and is adequate only in the smallest blood vessels (1–2 mm) (Fig. 18).

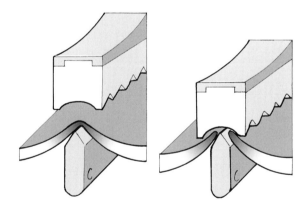

Fig. 18 When cutting tissue with the sharp blade of the shears, the lateral coagulation zone is 0.25 mm to 1 mm.

The blunt edge enables both coaptation and coagulation and, if desired, simultaneous cutting of tissue. Larger diameter blood vessels (2–3 mm) can be coagulated with this side of the blade (Fig. 19).

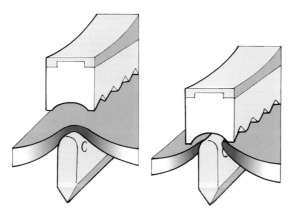

Fig. 19 When cutting tissue with the blunt blade of the shears, the lateral coagulation zone is 0.75 mm to 1.5 mm.

The flat edge is suitable for hemostasis by means of coagulation. It can coagulate vessels of up to 3 mm in diameter (Fig. 20).

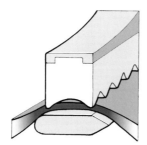

Fig. 20 During coagulation with the flat side, the zone of coagulation corresponds to the width of the tissue pad (2 mm) of the shears.

Cutting and coagulation ability of all the edges of the blade can be enhanced or decreased by:

- **The power level of the generator:** The higher the level, the more cutting and the less coagulation.
- **The grip force on the shears:** The stronger the force, the more cutting and the less coagulation.
- **The tension to the tissue:** The greater the tension, the more cutting and the less coagulation.
- **The application time of energy.**

The 5-mm shears are available in a length (35 cm) adequate for minimally invasive surgery and shorter lengths (14 cm, 23 cm) for open/conventional surgery.

The longer-length shears are available with either a straight or a curved active blade and pistol grip handle (Fig. 21).

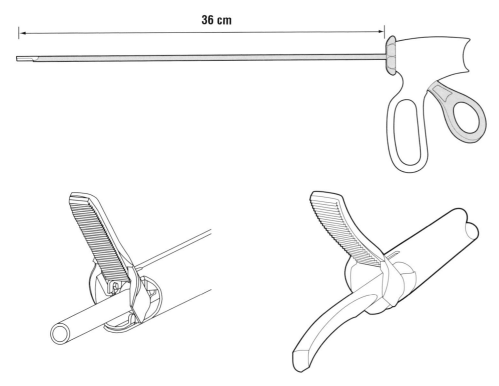

Fig. 21 5-mm Harmonic Scalpel shears for laparoscopic surgery.

The shorter shears are available only with a curved active blade and come with a scissor grip handle. The curved blade is designed to enhance visibility and access (Fig. 22).

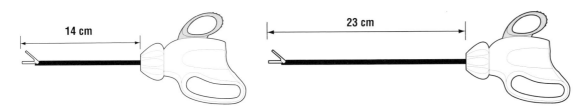

Fig. 22 5-mm Harmonic Scalpel shears for conventional/open surgery.

II

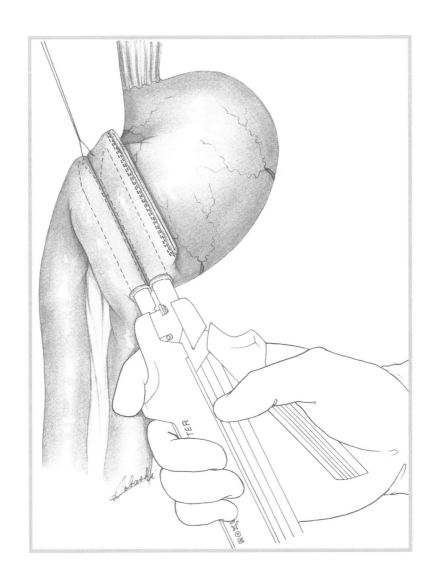

II

Surgical Procedures

1 Thoracic Surgery

Left Pneumonectomy

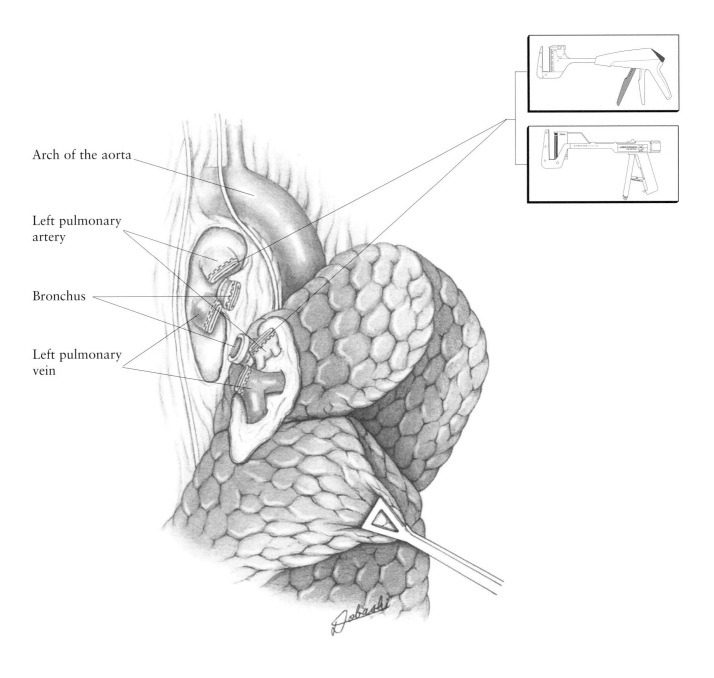

Arch of the aorta

Left pulmonary artery

Bronchus

Left pulmonary vein

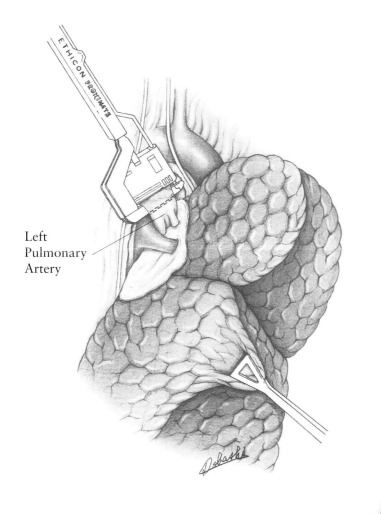

Left
Pulmonary
Artery

Once dissected, the pulmonary artery is
stapled using two firings of a vascular linear
stapler placed approximately 0.5 cm apart.

After the integrity of the staple lines has been
checked, the artery is transected between the
two lines of staples.

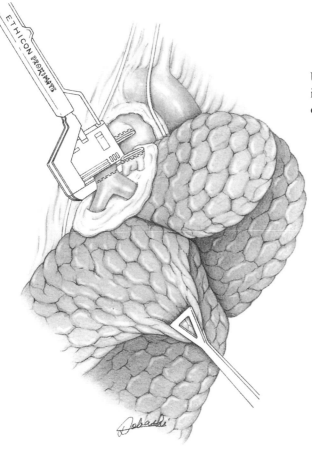

Using the same technique, the pulmonary vein is stapled and transected between the two rows of staples.

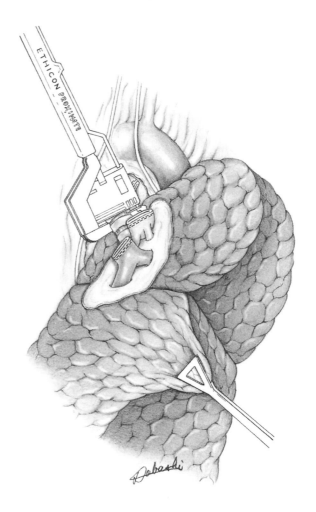

Once the main stem bronchus has been dissected, the linear stapler is positioned with the staples as close as possible to the tracheal carina, parallel to the cartilaginous rings. The bronchus is transected distal to the rows of staples.

Remove the specimen. The staple lines are carefully inspected for hemostasis and pneumostasis.

Lobectomy

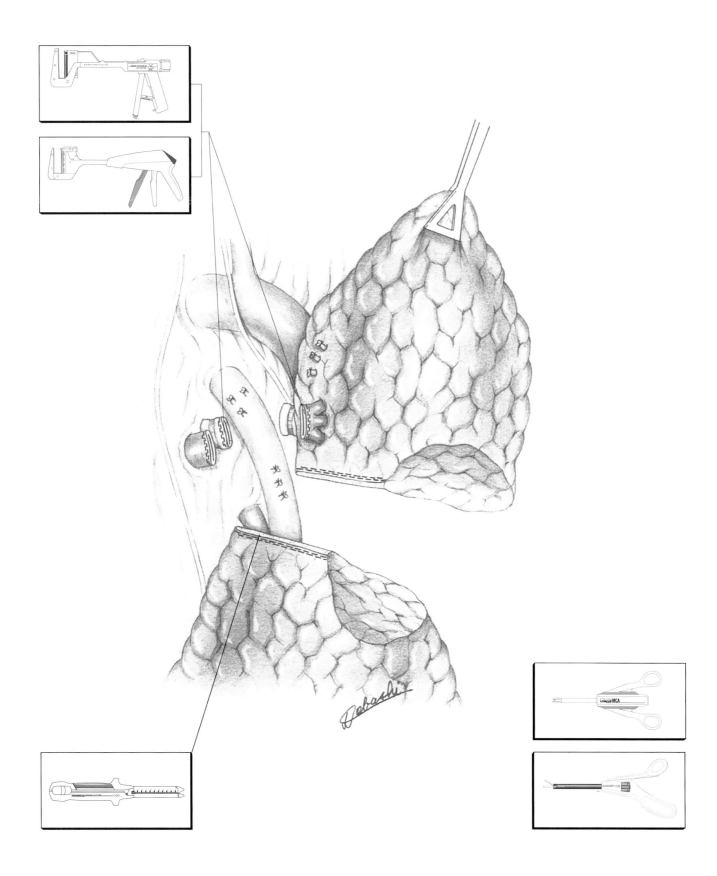

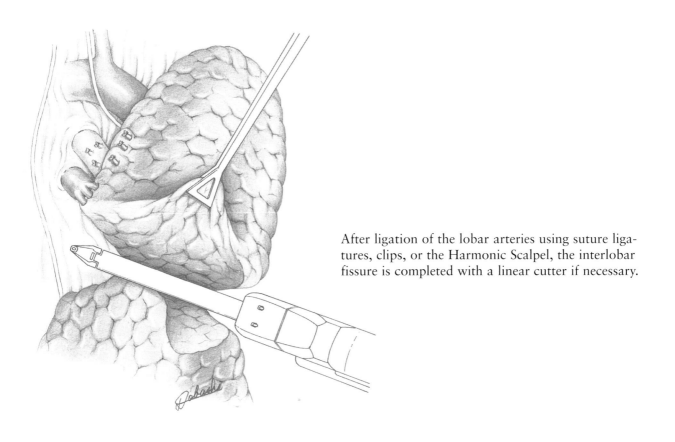

After ligation of the lobar arteries using suture ligatures, clips, or the Harmonic Scalpel, the interlobar fissure is completed with a linear cutter if necessary.

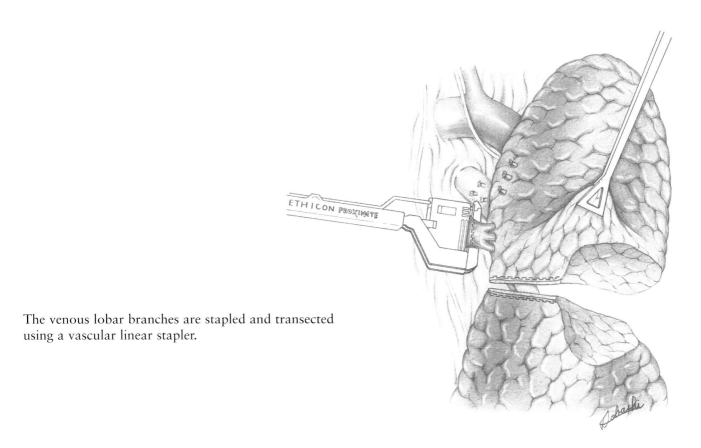

The venous lobar branches are stapled and transected using a vascular linear stapler.

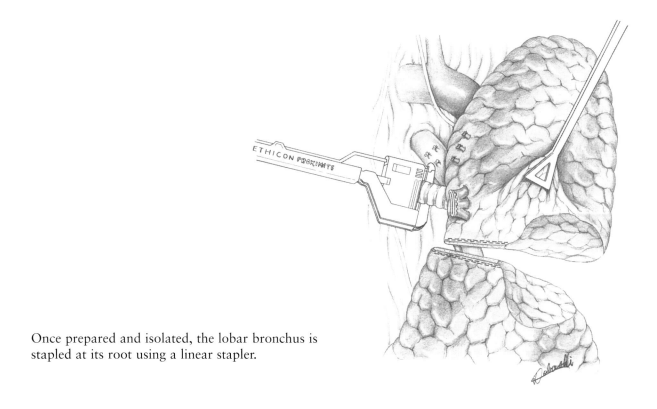

Once prepared and isolated, the lobar bronchus is stapled at its root using a linear stapler.

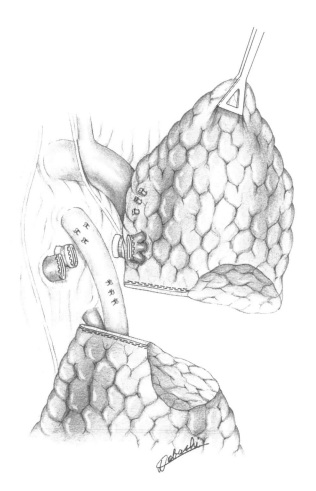

The lobar bronchus is transected distal to the line of staples and the specimen is removed. The staple lines are carefully inspected for hemostasis and pneumostasis.

Atypical/Non-Anatomic Resections (Apical Resection)

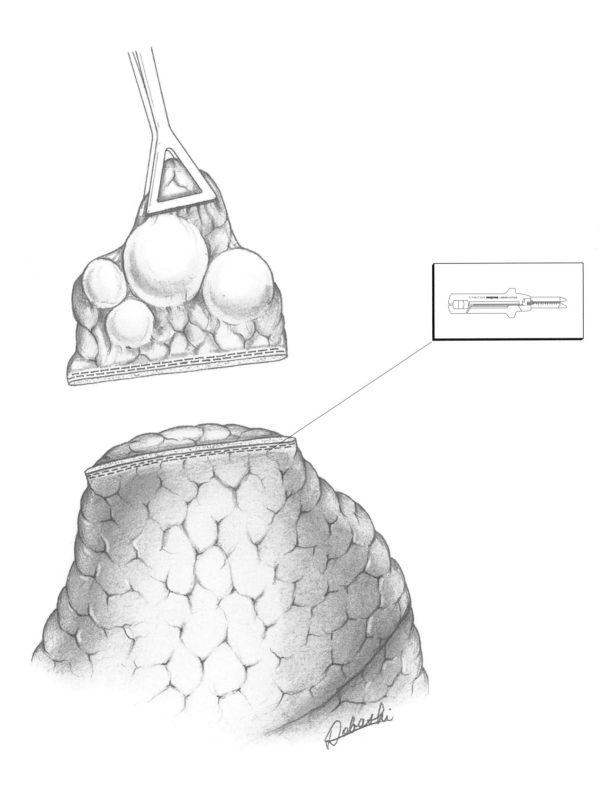

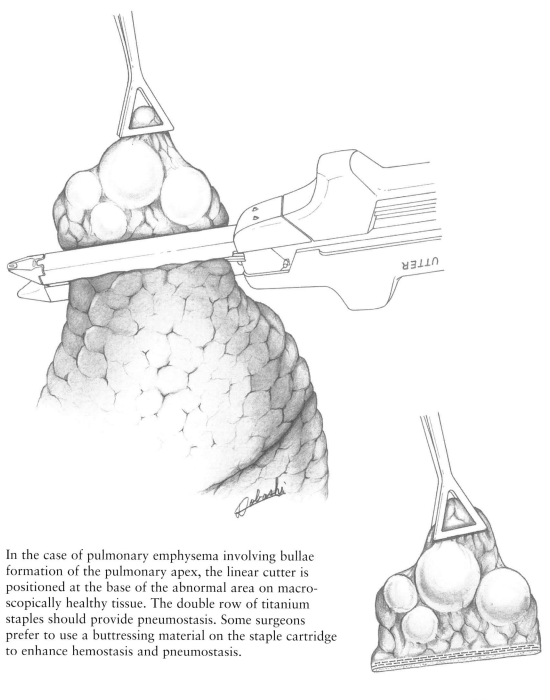

In the case of pulmonary emphysema involving bullae formation of the pulmonary apex, the linear cutter is positioned at the base of the abnormal area on macroscopically healthy tissue. The double row of titanium staples should provide pneumostasis. Some surgeons prefer to use a buttressing material on the staple cartridge to enhance hemostasis and pneumostasis.

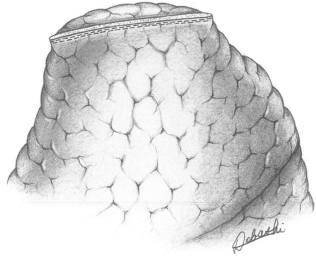

The staple lines are carefully inspected for hemostasis and pneumostasis.

Atypical/Non-Anatomic Resections (Wedge Resection)

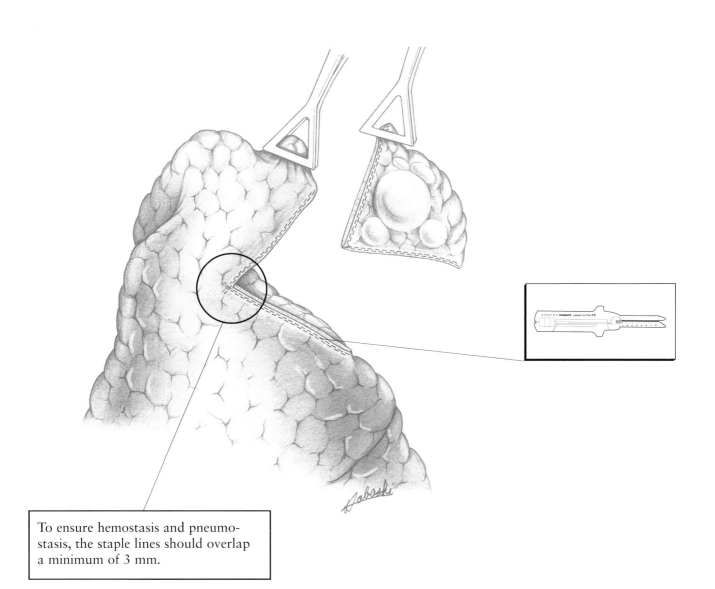

To ensure hemostasis and pneumostasis, the staple lines should overlap
a minimum of 3 mm.

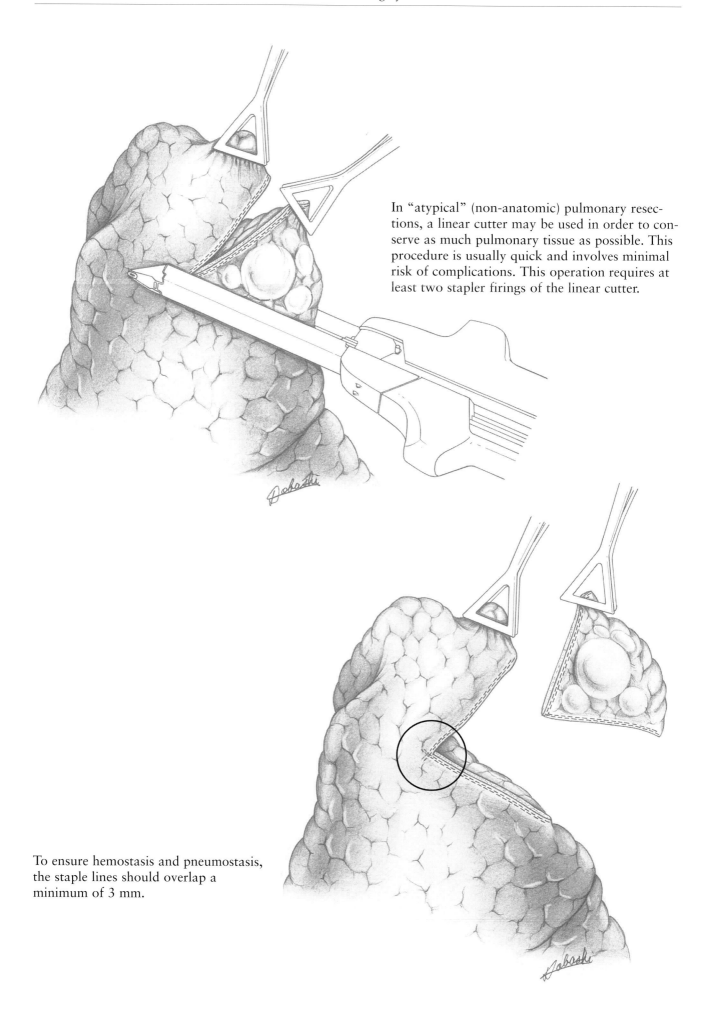

In "atypical" (non-anatomic) pulmonary resections, a linear cutter may be used in order to conserve as much pulmonary tissue as possible. This procedure is usually quick and involves minimal risk of complications. This operation requires at least two stapler firings of the linear cutter.

To ensure hemostasis and pneumostasis, the staple lines should overlap a minimum of 3 mm.

2 Esophageal Surgery

Zenker's Diverticulum

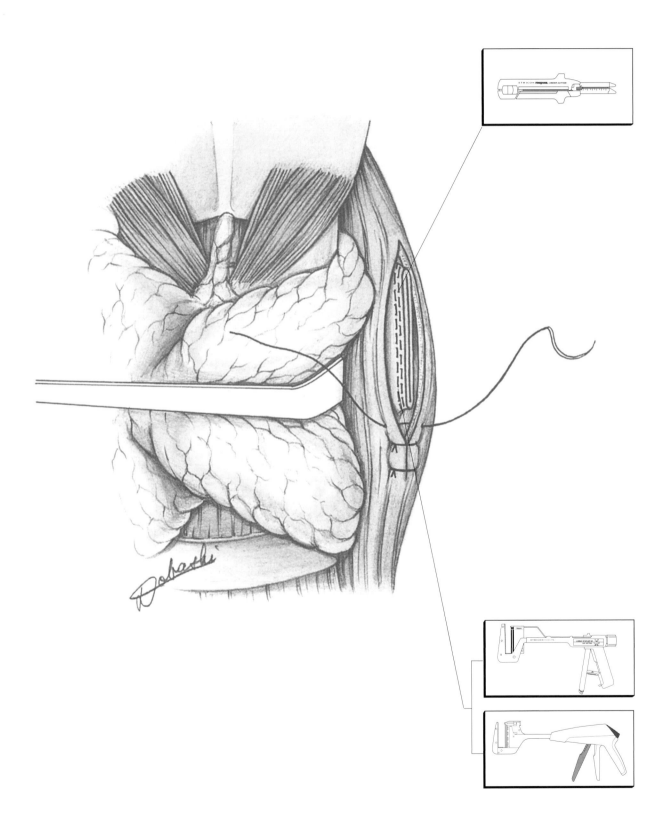

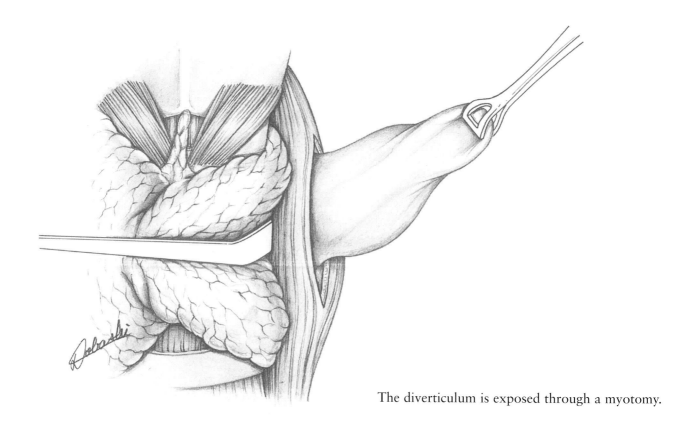

The diverticulum is exposed through a myotomy.

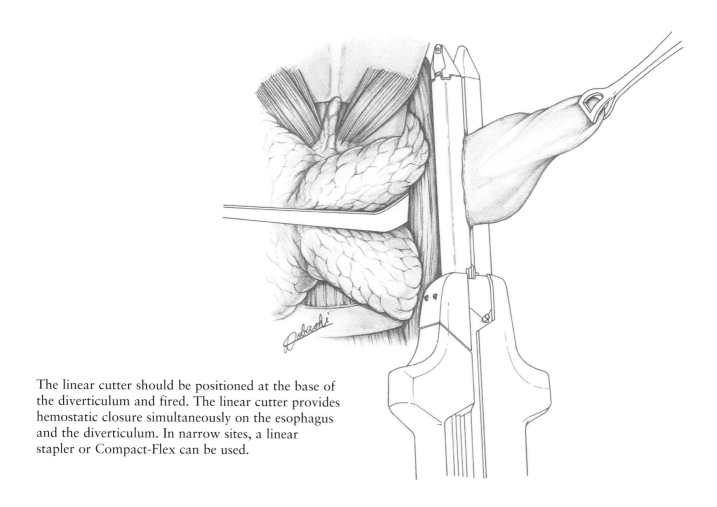

The linear cutter should be positioned at the base of
the diverticulum and fired. The linear cutter provides
hemostatic closure simultaneously on the esophagus
and the diverticulum. In narrow sites, a linear
stapler or Compact-Flex can be used.

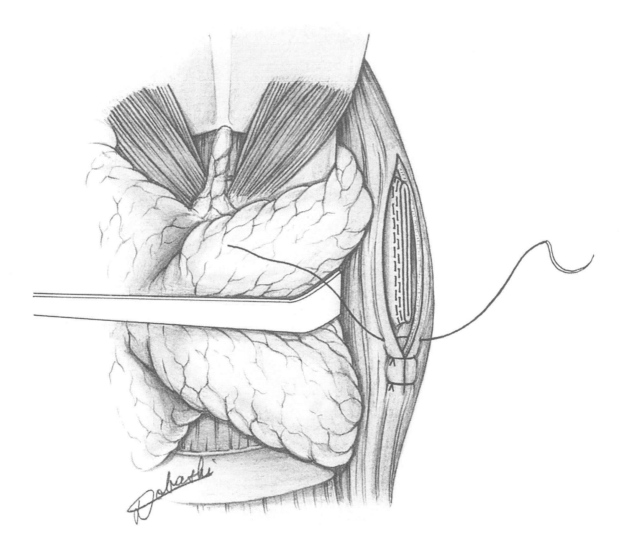

The myotomy is closed by manual suturing.

Reconstruction of the Thoracic Esophagus

Esophagectomy, Gastric Tube, and Cervical Anastomosis

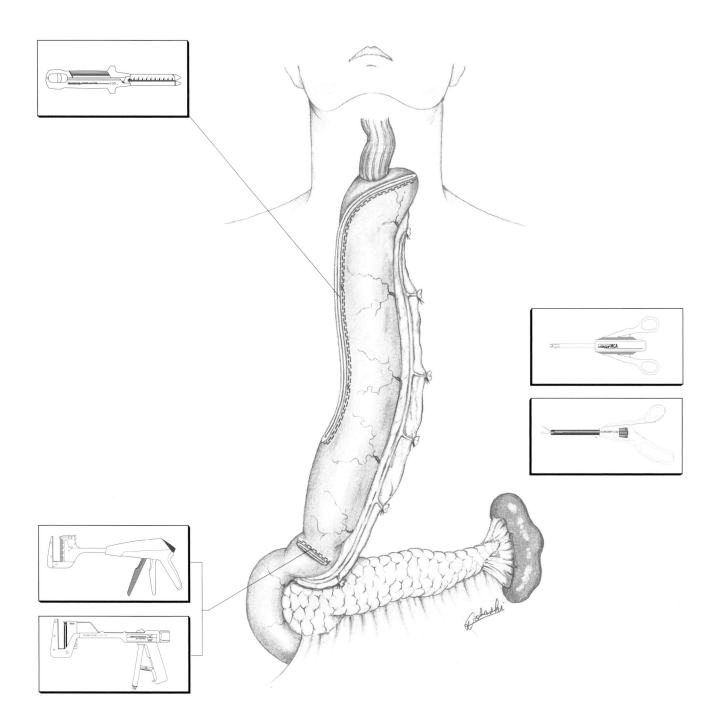

Reconstruction of the thoracic esophagus with a gastric tube and a cervical anastomosis can be performed through a right thoracotomy in combination with abdominal and cervical incisions, or utilizing a transhiatal approach, thus avoiding a thoracotomy.

Advanced laparoscopic techniques can be utilized in both the abdominal and thoracic dissections.
The anastomosis can then be performed through a separate cervical incision.

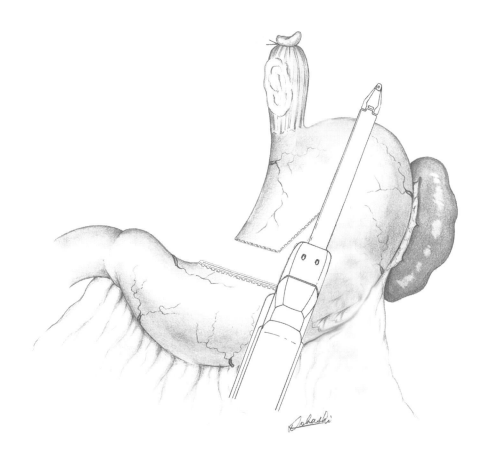

After the thoracic portion of the operation is completed, whether performed using an open procedure or with a thoracoscope, the abdominal portion is performed with the patient in the supine position. The stomach is mobilized using suture ligatures, clips, or the Harmonic Scalpel. The gastric tube is completed with several applications of the linear cutter, starting from the level of the fifth branch of the right gastric artery.

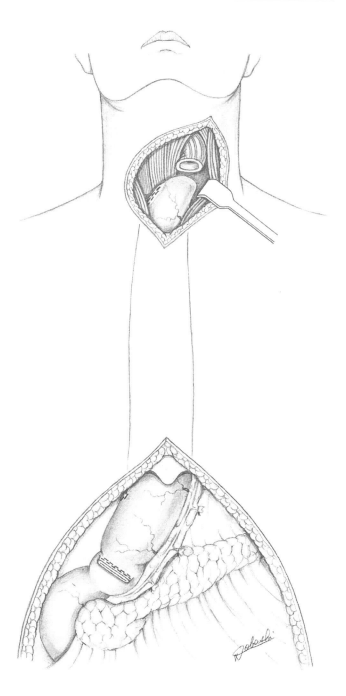

A pyloroplasty is performed with a linear stapler or sutures. The gastric tube is delivered to the neck by gentle traction on the specimen from the cervical incision and gentle pressure from below. The pylorus will be located 2 cm below the hiatus. Performing an esophagogastrostomy manually creates the cervical portion of the reconstruction. After ensuring that the anastomosis has been satisfactorily performed, the surgeon closes the incisions.

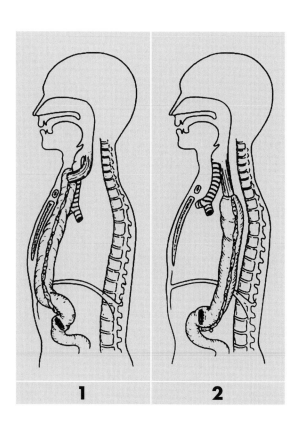

1   **2**

The substitute can be positioned substernally (1) or anatomically (2), the latter being the most common practice.

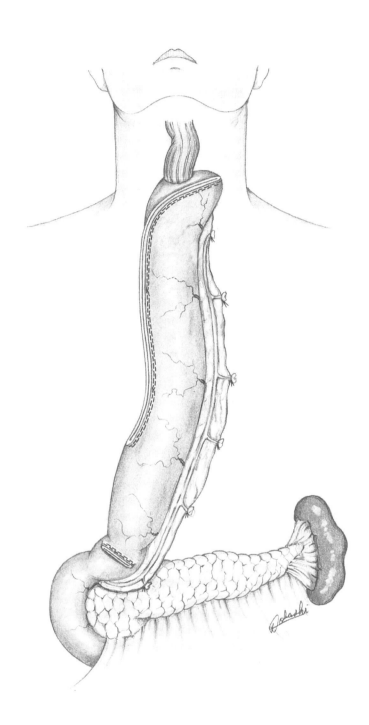

Completed esophageal reconstruction with an
end-to-side esophagogastric anastomosis.

Reconstruction of the Thoracic Esophagus

Esophagectomy, Colon Replacement, and Cervical Anastomosis

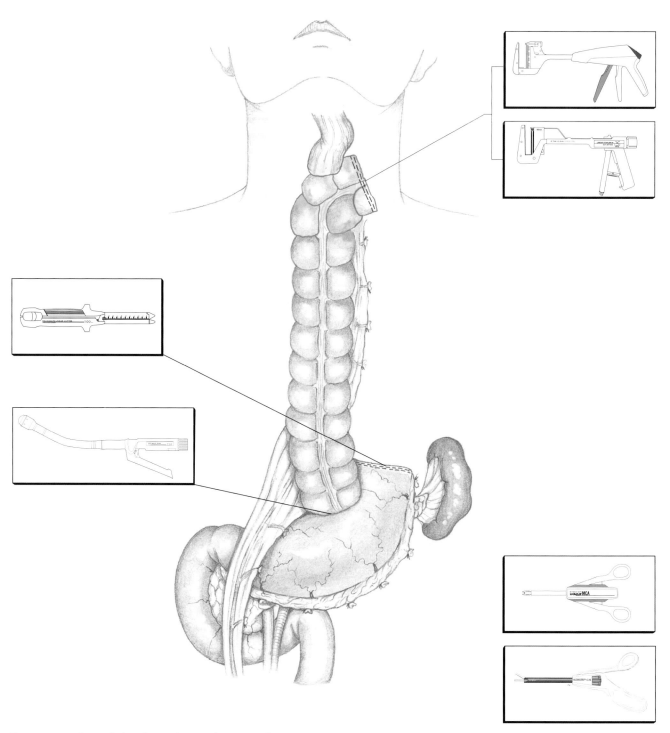

Reconstruction of the thoracic esophagus utilizing
the transverse colon.

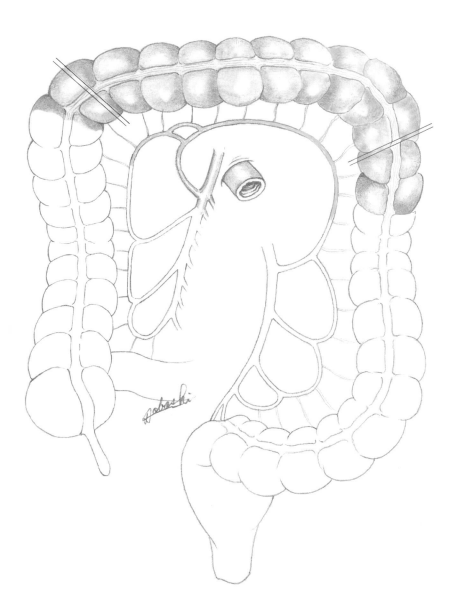

The transverse colon is used in the majority of cases.
The use of the right colon is possible, but the volume of
the cecum may be too great for the retrosternal space.
Attention must be paid to the selection and mobilization
of the segment of colon to be used for the reconstruction.
The selected segment should be of sufficient length to
allow a tension-free anastomosis and have favorable
vascular anatomy, which will allow for adequate arterial
blood supply and venous drainage following mobilization.
A linear cutter is used to create the lines of transection
shown above.

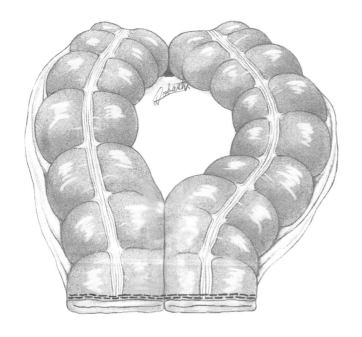

A functional end-to-end anastomosis is performed between the right and left colon with a linear cutter in order to reestablish intestinal continuity. See pages 213 and 214 for a detailed description of this technique.

A cervical end-to-side anastomosis is performed with hand sutures.

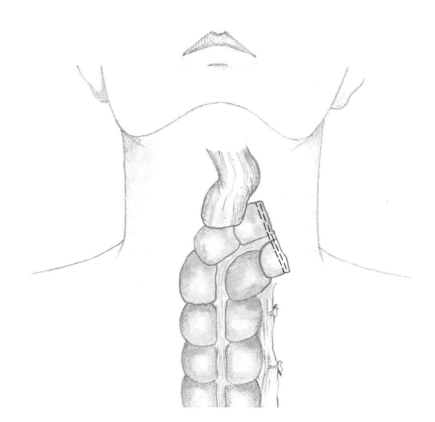

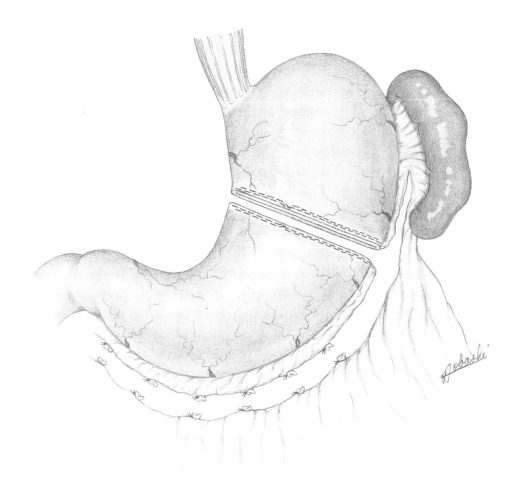

After the inferior portion of the stomach has been mobilized using
suture ligatures, clips, or the Harmonic Scalpel, a proximal
gastrectomy is performed using a linear cutter. In doing this,
the spleen is routinely preserved.

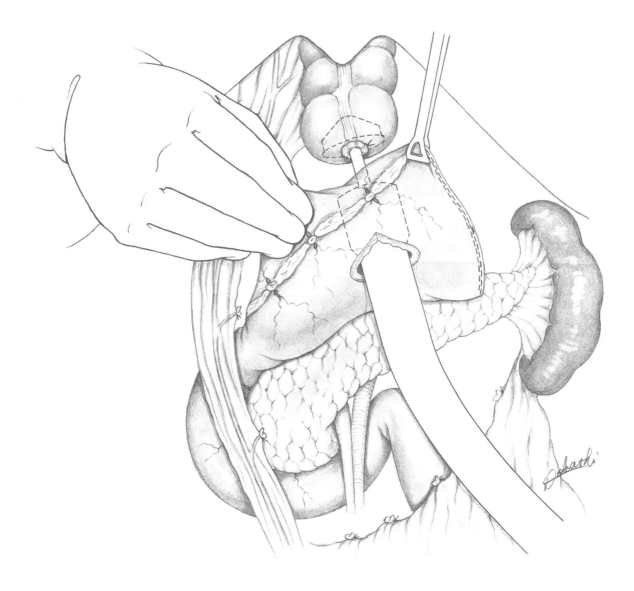

To perform the cologastric anastomosis, a purse-string
suture is placed in the distal transverse colon, and the
anvil of the circular stapler is inserted. The purse-string
suture is tied around the anvil center rod. A gastrotomy is
created for the insertion of the circular stapler. The anvil
is attached to the integral trocar and the circular stapler is
closed and fired, creating the cologastic anastomosis.
After the circular stapler is withdrawn, the integrity of
the tissue donuts should be examined. If donuts are not
complete, the anastomosis should be carefully checked for
leakage and appropriate repairs made. The cologastric
anastomosis is made about a third of the way down from
the gastric fundus. Here, the anastomosis is performed on
the anterior wall, leaving at least 3 cm between the linear
cutter and the circular staple lines. A common technique
is to advance the colon with its vascular pedicle posterior
to the stomach. The illustrations on pages 92 and 93
demonstrate an alternate technique, in which prior
pyloroplasty is covered by the vascular pedicle of the
transverse colon.

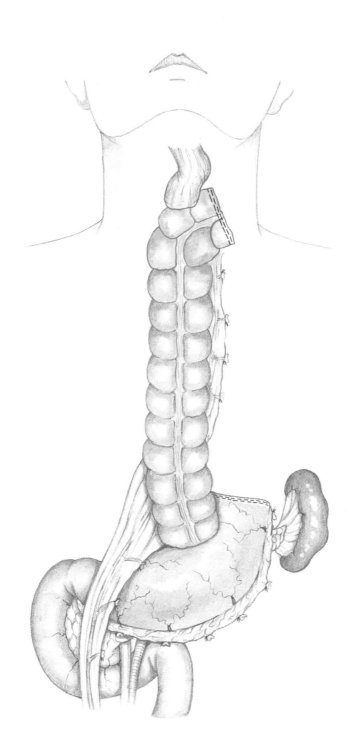

The completed cologastric anastomosis.

Reconstruction of the Thoracic Esophagus

Esophagectomy with Thoracic Anastomosis: The Ivor Lewis Procedure

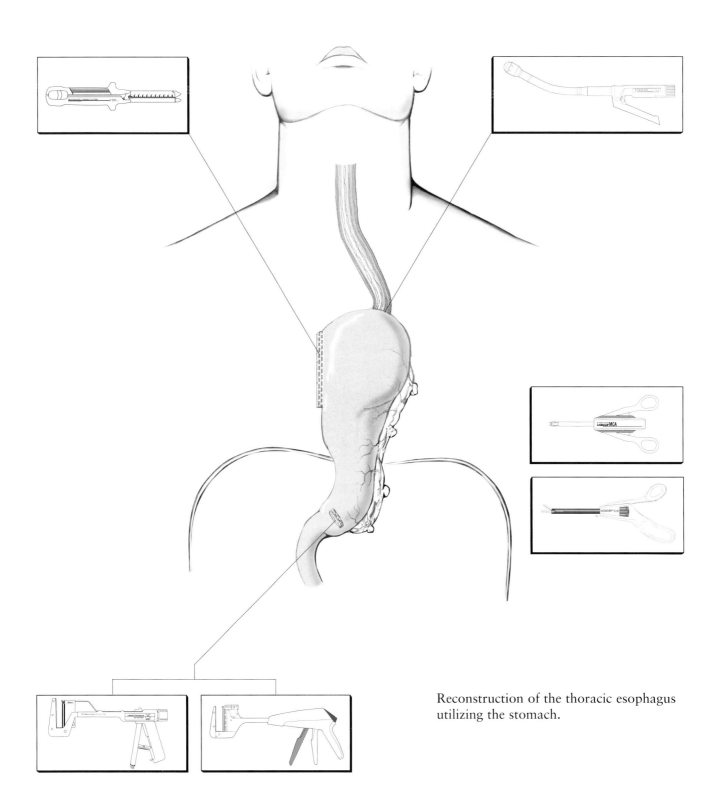

Reconstruction of the thoracic esophagus utilizing the stomach.

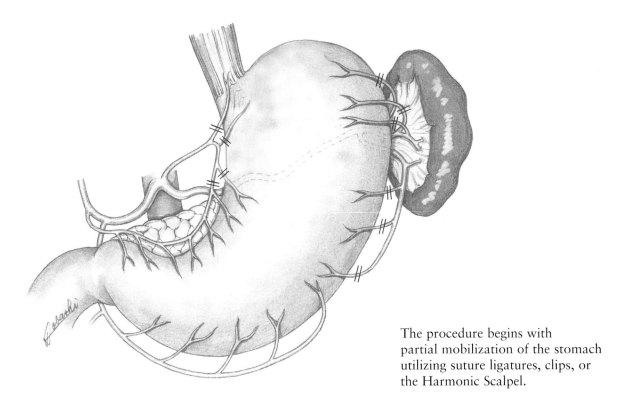

The procedure begins with partial mobilization of the stomach utilizing suture ligatures, clips, or the Harmonic Scalpel.

As a result of the transection of the vagal nerve trunks, a pyloroplasty should be performed. This can be accomplished with a linear stapler in a later step of the procedure.

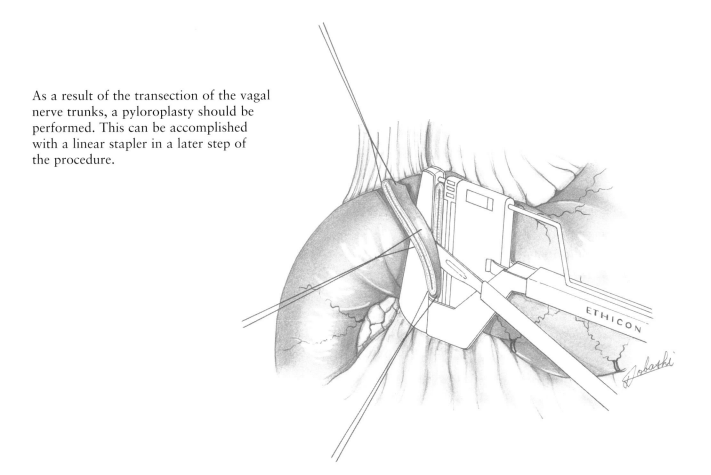

Thoracic portion of the procedure

After the esophagus has been transected proximal to the diseased area, a purse-string suture is placed at its distal end. In order to place an adequate purse-string suture, the mucosa of the esophagus is exteriorized with four graspers. In fashioning the purse-string, special attention must be paid so that all layers of the esophageal wall are included

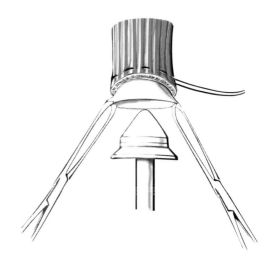

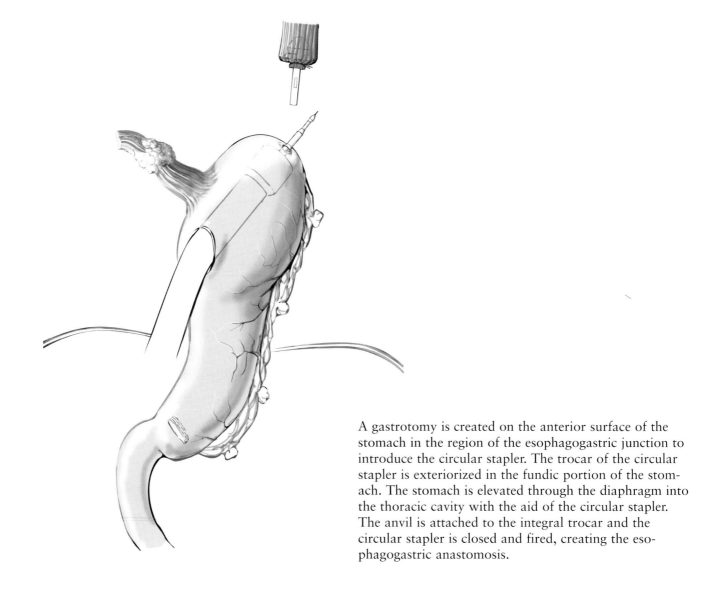

A gastrotomy is created on the anterior surface of the stomach in the region of the esophagogastric junction to introduce the circular stapler. The trocar of the circular stapler is exteriorized in the fundic portion of the stomach. The stomach is elevated through the diaphragm into the thoracic cavity with the aid of the circular stapler. The anvil is attached to the integral trocar and the circular stapler is closed and fired, creating the esophagogastric anastomosis.

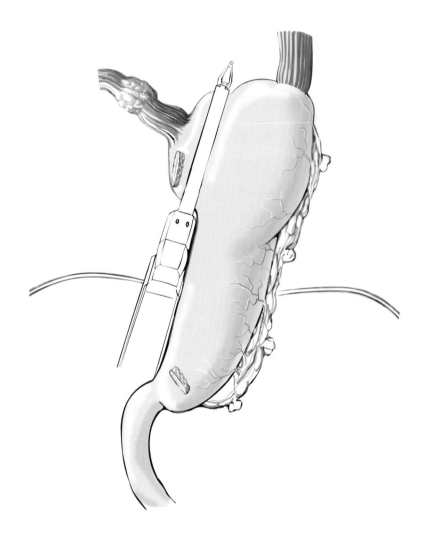

After the circular stapler is withdrawn, the tissue
donuts should be examined for completeness.
The donuts should be intact and include all tissue
layers. If the donuts are not complete, the anastomosis should be carefully checked for leakage
and appropriate repairs made. The gastric tube is
created with a linear cutter or linear stapler, removing the gastrotomy with the specimen. A distance
of 3 cm must be maintained between the two staple
lines.

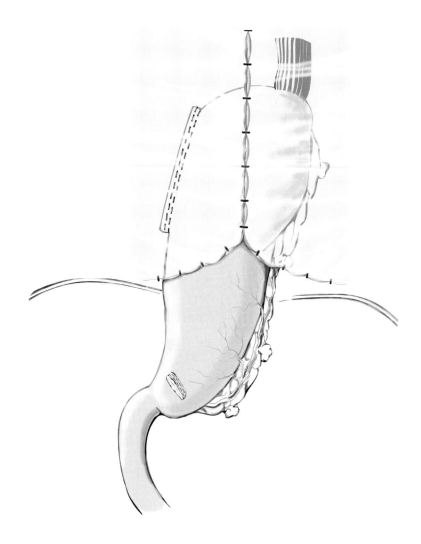

The basic principle in performing an anastomosis is to avoid tension between the two segments. The weight of the stomach, when suspended only by the staples of the anastomosis, may cause tension on the anastomosis and contribute to anastomotic leakage. To avoid this traction on the staple line, the top of the gastric tube is suspended from the margins of the mediastinal pleura.

The anastomosis is then buried under a flap of the mediastinal pleura. This will reduce the risk of mediastinal contamination in the case of anastomotic leakage.

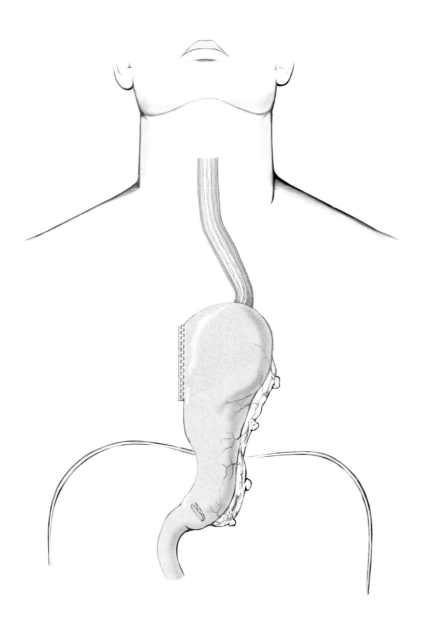

View of the completed intrathoracic esophagogastric anastomosis.

Reconstruction of the Thoracic Esophagus

Distal Esophagectomy and Total Gastrectomy with Jejunum Replacement and Thoracic Anastomosis

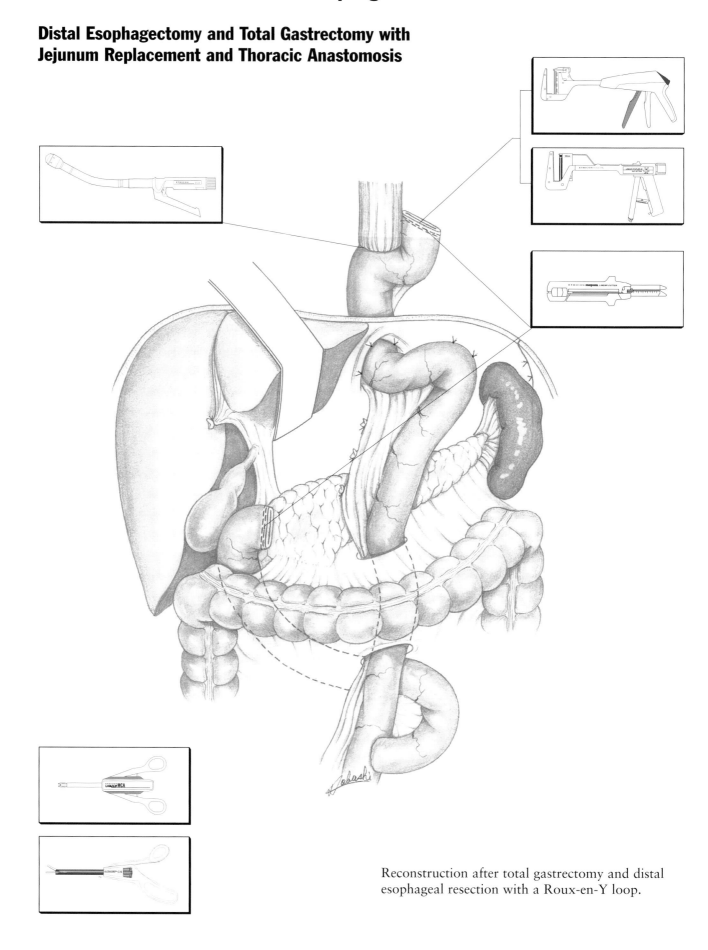

Reconstruction after total gastrectomy and distal esophageal resection with a Roux-en-Y loop.

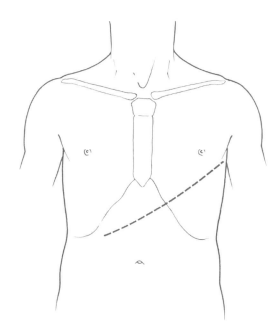

The operation is performed through a left combined thoracoabdominal incision with the patient's left side elevated about 45°.

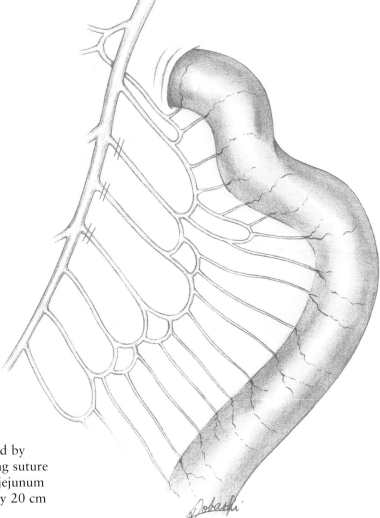

A 50-cm retrocolic Roux-en-Y loop is prepared by ligating a portion of at least three arcades using suture ligatures, clips, or the Harmonic Scalpel. The jejunum is transected with a linear cutter approximately 20 cm distal to the ligament of Treitz.

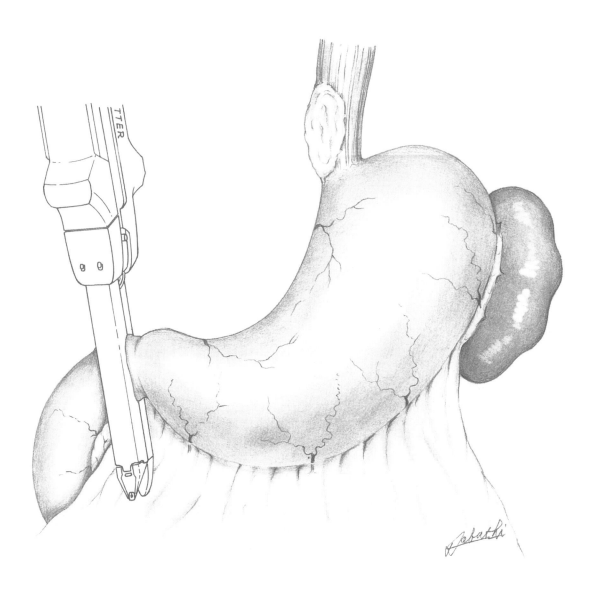

The stomach, including the omentum, is mobilized using suture ligatures, clips, or the Harmonic Scalpel and transected 2 cm distal to the pylorus with a linear cutter or linear stapler. The advantage of the linear cutter is that it simultaneously cuts and staples, thus avoiding spillage. The linear stapler, however, is easier to position without tension on the tissue.

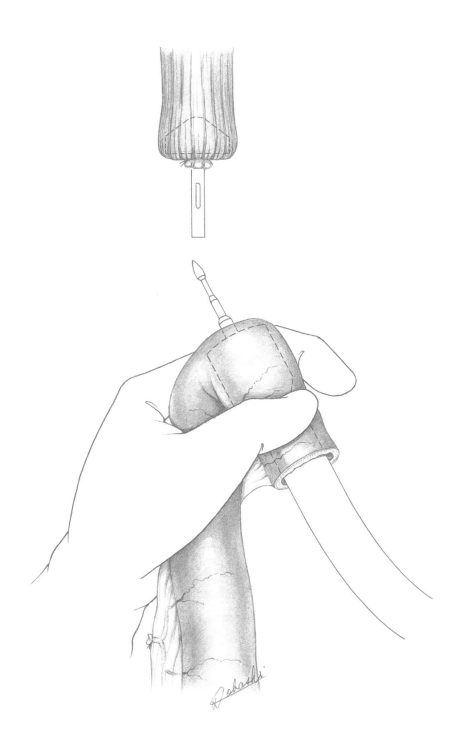

After the esophagus has been transected proximal to the diseased area, the specimen is removed. A purse-string suture is then placed on the distal end of the remaining esophagus. The anvil of the circular stapler is introduced into the esophagus and the purse-string suture tied. The circular stapler is inserted through the open proximal end of the distal jejunal segment, and the integral trocar is advanced to pierce its antimesenteric wall 5 cm from the open end.

The anvil is attached to the integral trocar and the circular stapler is closed and fired, creating the esophagojejunostomy. After the circular stapler is withdrawn, the tissue donuts are examined for completeness. The donuts should be intact and include all tissue layers. If the donuts are not complete, the anastomosis should be carefully checked for leakage and appropriate repairs made.

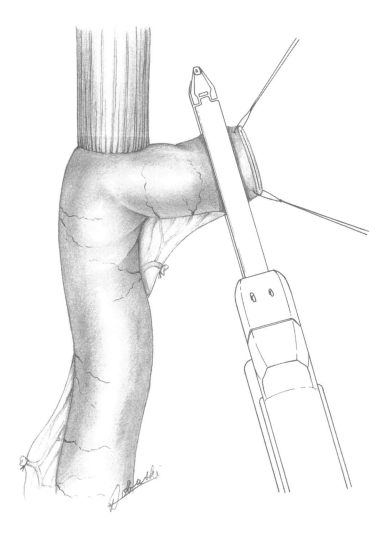

The open end of the jejunal loop is closed using a linear cutter or linear stapler.

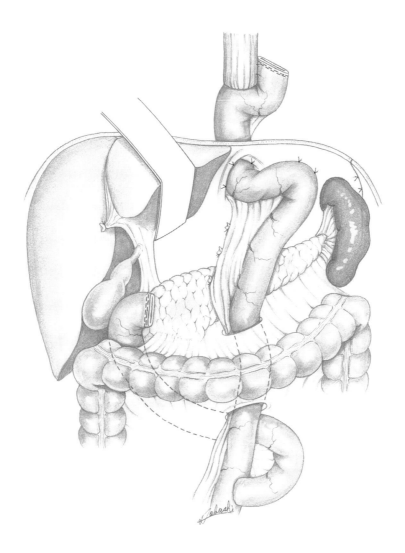

An end-to-side jejunojejunostomy is performed to create the Roux-en-Y loop. The jejunal interposition segment should be fixed to the diaphragm and hiatus to avoid tension on the proximal anastomosis. Attachment of the blind end of the jejunal loop to the esophagus is seldom necessary.

Ligation of Esophageal Varices

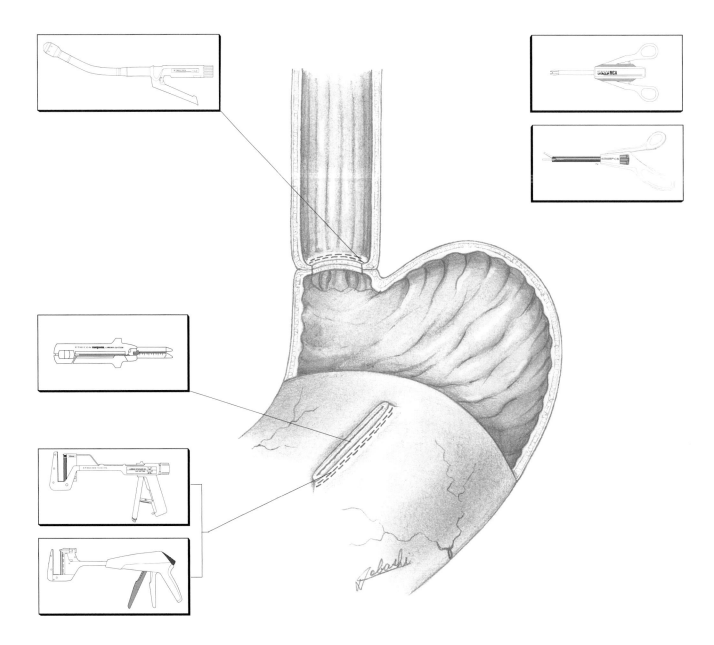

Minimal esophageal resection utilizing a circular stapling
device for esophageal varices.

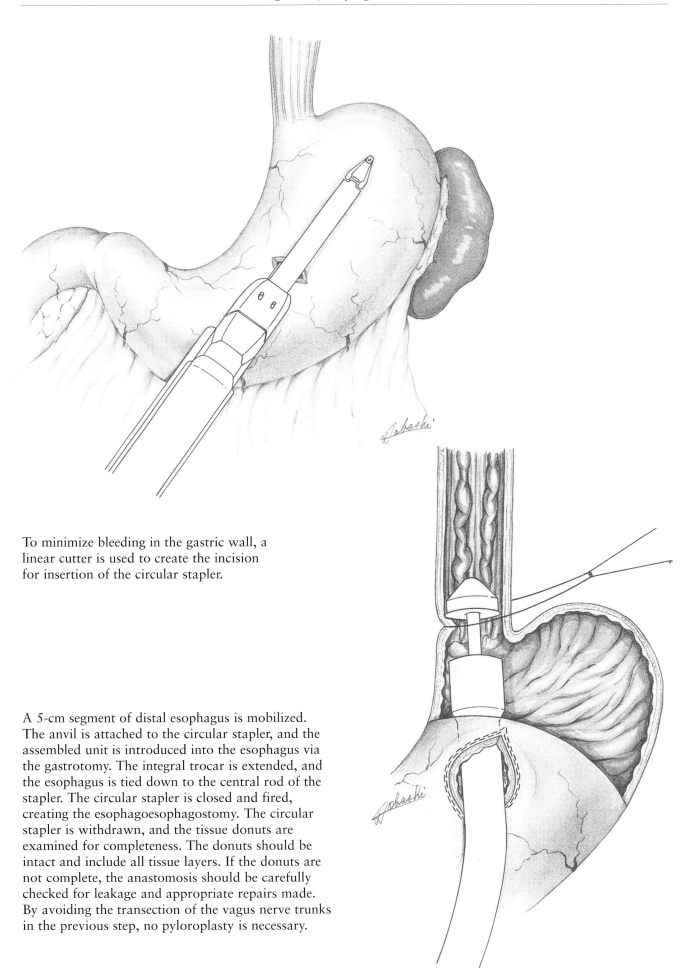

To minimize bleeding in the gastric wall, a linear cutter is used to create the incision for insertion of the circular stapler.

A 5-cm segment of distal esophagus is mobilized. The anvil is attached to the circular stapler, and the assembled unit is introduced into the esophagus via the gastrotomy. The integral trocar is extended, and the esophagus is tied down to the central rod of the stapler. The circular stapler is closed and fired, creating the esophagoesophagostomy. The circular stapler is withdrawn, and the tissue donuts are examined for completeness. The donuts should be intact and include all tissue layers. If the donuts are not complete, the anastomosis should be carefully checked for leakage and appropriate repairs made. By avoiding the transection of the vagus nerve trunks in the previous step, no pyloroplasty is necessary.

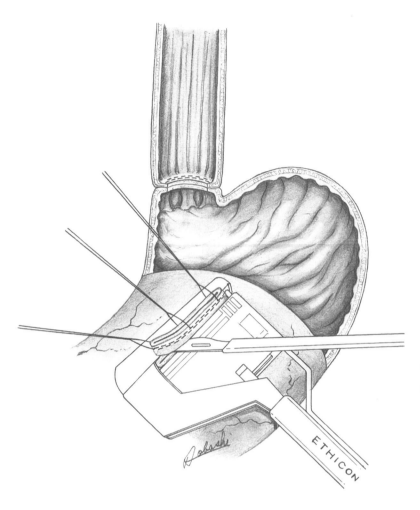

The gastrotomy is closed using a linear stapler or hand sutures.

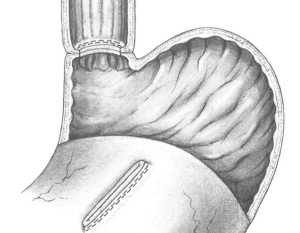

The completed ligation of esophageal varicosities.

3 Gastric Surgery

Gastrostomy

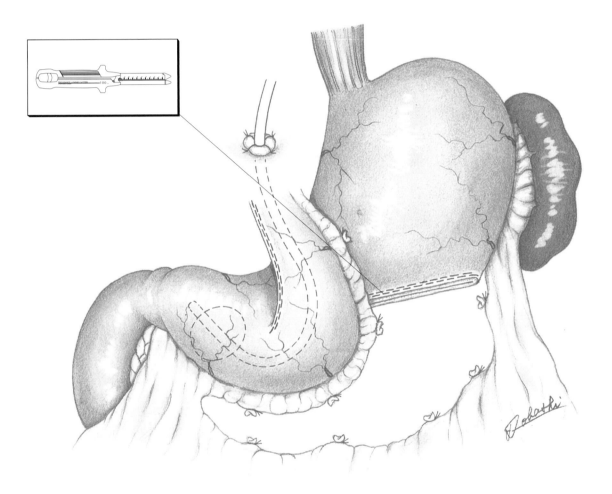

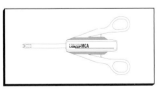

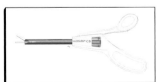

Gastrostomy performed utilizing a linear cutter.

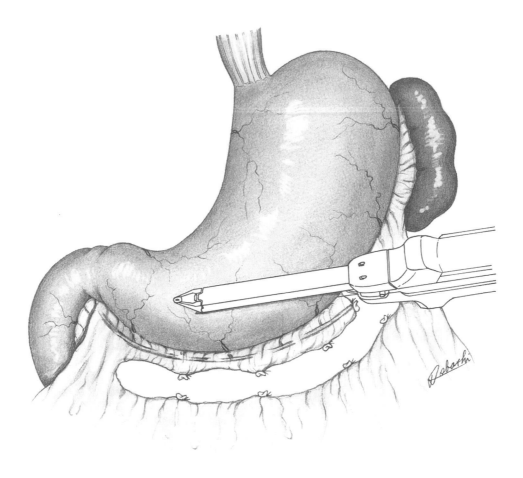

Partial mobilization of the stomach along the greater
curvature is performed using suture ligatures, clips, or the
Harmonic Scalpel. The alimentary tube is created with the
linear cutter.

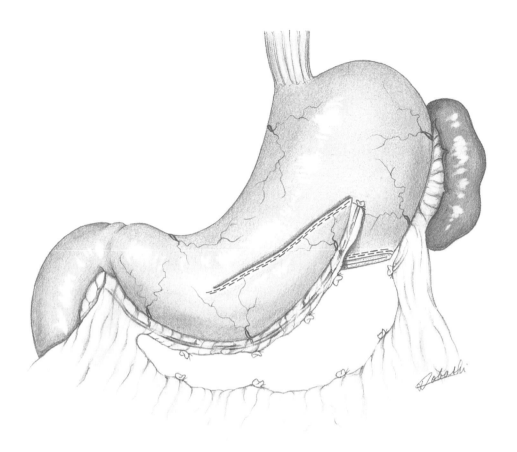

Here are examples of different variations in creating the gastric tube. In constructing the tube, special attention must be paid to its diameter so that it properly accommodates a feeding tube.

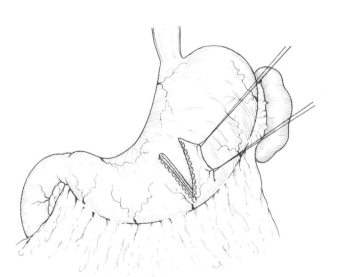

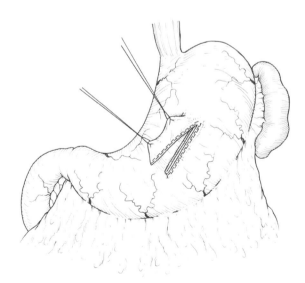

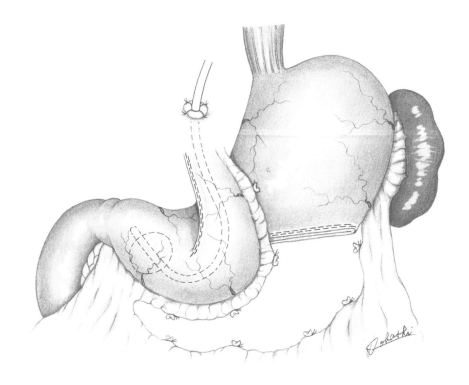

The procedure is completed by creating a small stab incision in the abdominal wall. The newly created gastric tube is secured to the skin with sutures. The tip of the tube is amputated to create the alimentary opening. This opening should be just large enough to accommodate a feeding tube.

Partial Gastrectomy

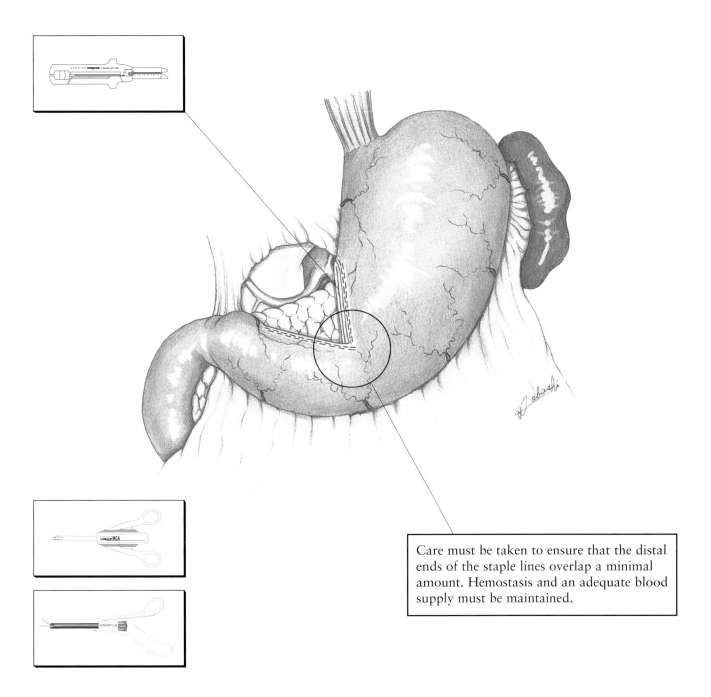

Care must be taken to ensure that the distal ends of the staple lines overlap a minimal amount. Hemostasis and an adequate blood supply must be maintained.

The main indication for the so-called wedge resection is found in ulcer surgery.

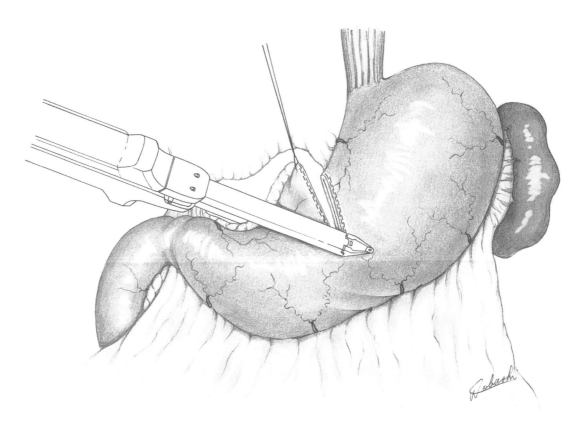

Partial mobilization of the stomach along the lesser curvature
is performed using suture ligatures, clips, or the Harmonic
Scalpel. A partial resection of the stomach is performed by
firing the linear cutter twice.

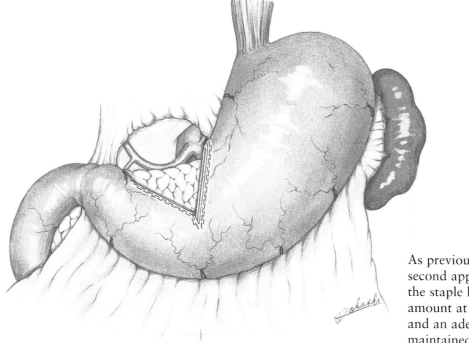

As previously mentioned, during the
second application of the linear cutter,
the staple lines must overlap a minimal
amount at their distal ends. Hemostasis
and an adequate blood supply must be
maintained.

Billroth I

Subtotal Gastrectomy with a Side-to-End Gastroduodenostomy

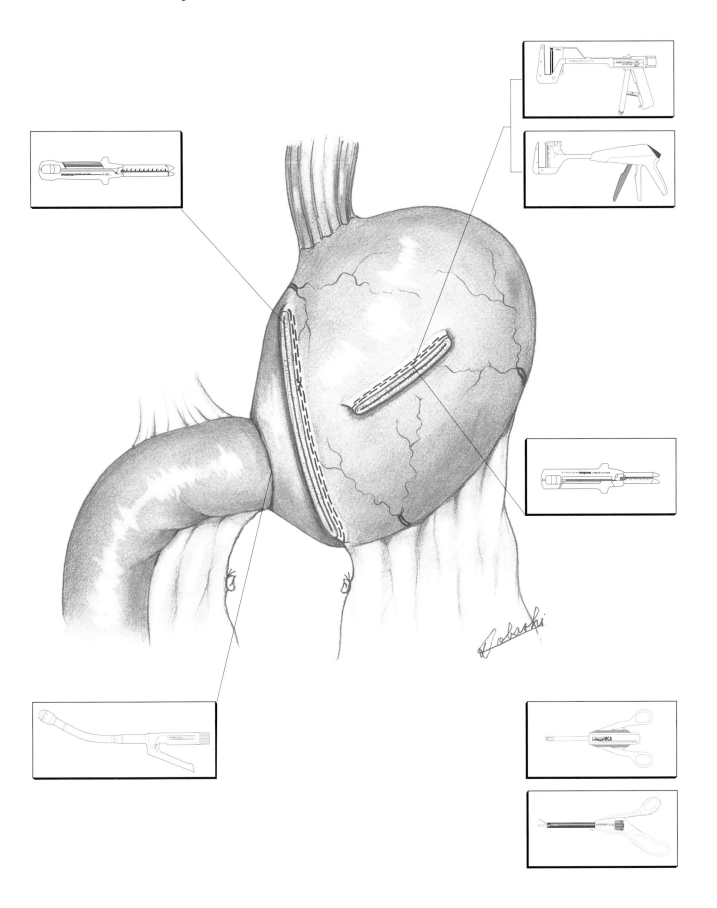

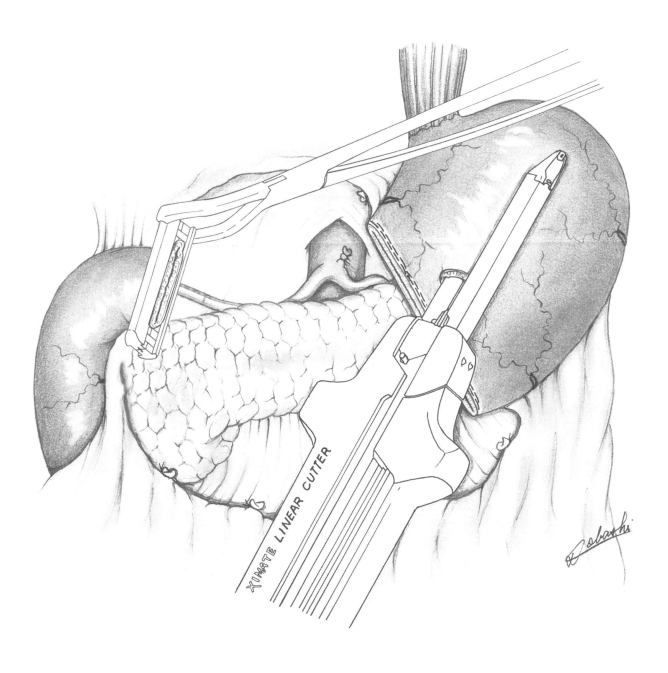

The procedure begins with mobilization of the stomach using suture ligatures, clips, or the Harmonic Scalpel. A distal subtotal gastrectomy is performed with two firings of the linear cutter. The duodenal staple line is excised, and a purse-string suture is placed. A small gastrotomy is performed at least 3 cm from the proximal staple line to permit the insertion of the forks of the linear cutter. The linear cutter is fired to create a gastrotomy large enough to allow the introduction of a circular stapler.

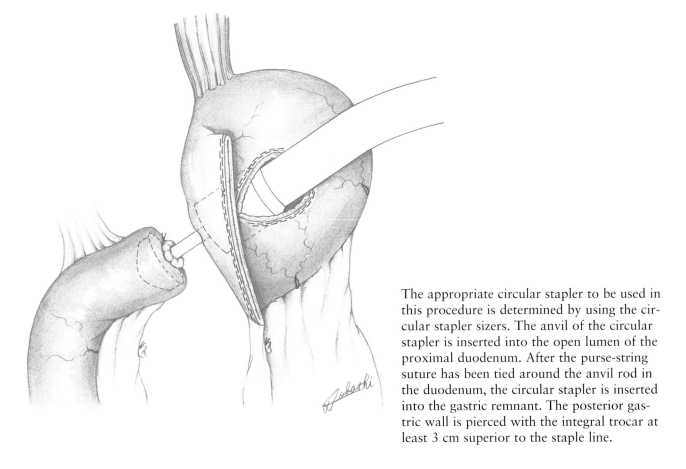

The appropriate circular stapler to be used in this procedure is determined by using the circular stapler sizers. The anvil of the circular stapler is inserted into the open lumen of the proximal duodenum. After the purse-string suture has been tied around the anvil rod in the duodenum, the circular stapler is inserted into the gastric remnant. The posterior gastric wall is pierced with the integral trocar at least 3 cm superior to the staple line.

The instrument head and anvil center rod are connected, and the instrument is fired to create a side-to-end gastro-duodenostomy. The staple line is examined for hemostasis and proper staple closure. After the circular stapler is withdrawn, the tissue donuts are examined for completeness. If the donuts are not complete, the anastomosis should be carefully checked for leakage and appropriate repairs made.

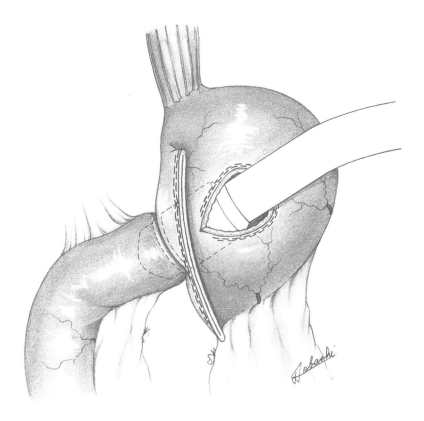

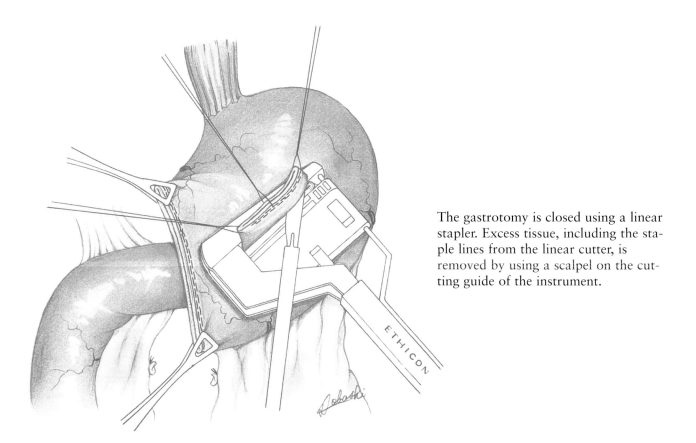

The gastrotomy is closed using a linear stapler. Excess tissue, including the staple lines from the linear cutter, is removed by using a scalpel on the cutting guide of the instrument.

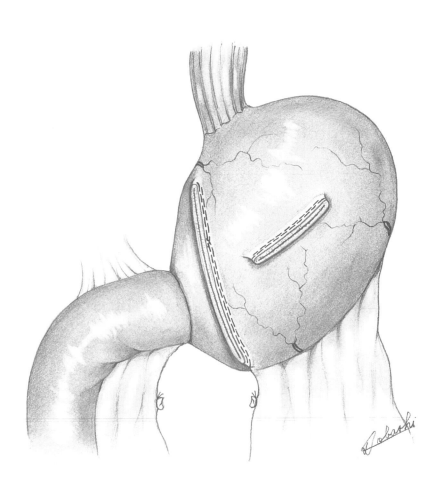

Completed gastroduodenostomy.

Billroth I

Subtotal Gastrectomy with End-to-End Gastroduodenostomy

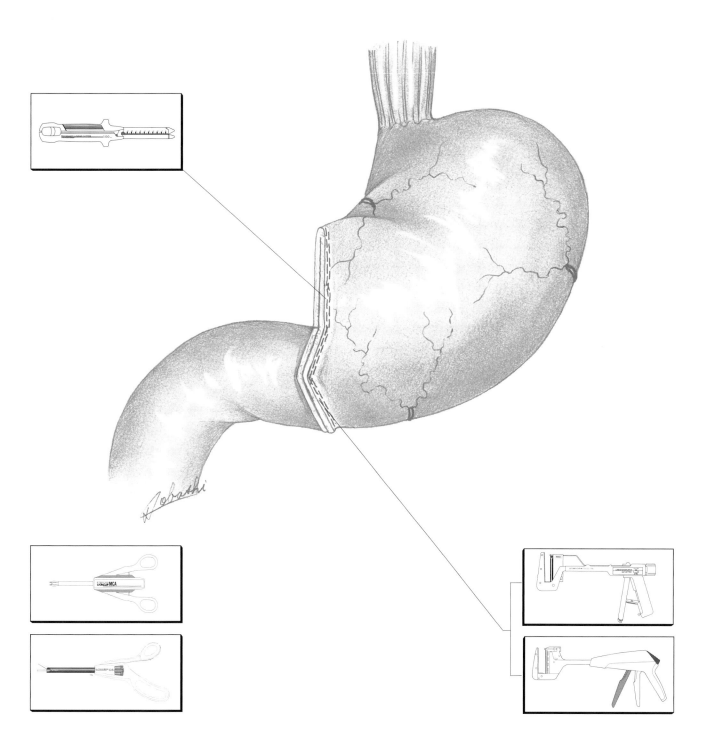

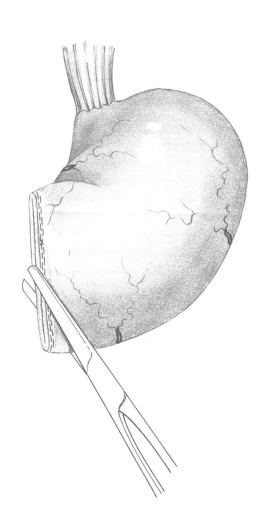

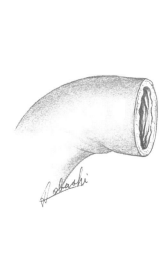

The procedure begins with mobilization of the stomach using
suture ligatures, clips, or the Harmonic Scalpel. A distal subtotal
gastrectomy is performed with two firings of a linear cutter. The
distal staple line at the duodenum is excised. The lower third of
the staple line of the remaining stomach is resected with scissors.
Care must be taken to ensure that the lumen of the gastric
opening and the duodenum are aligned and of equal size.

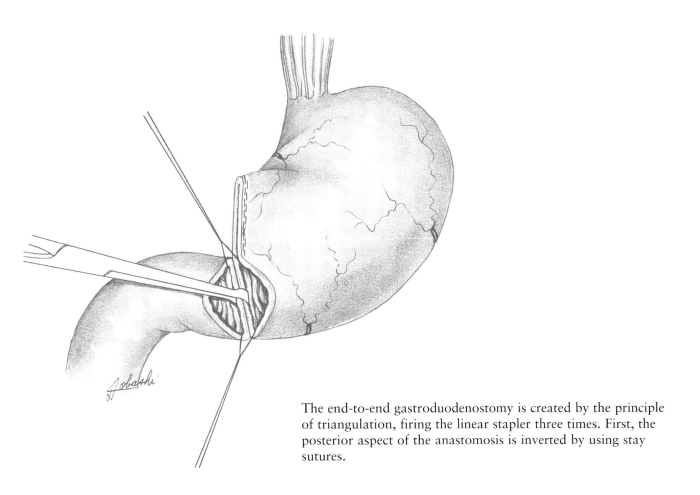

The end-to-end gastroduodenostomy is created by the principle of triangulation, firing the linear stapler three times. First, the posterior aspect of the anastomosis is inverted by using stay sutures.

A linear stapler is used to create the posterior aspect of the anastomosis. After the instrument is fired, the excess tissue should be excised.

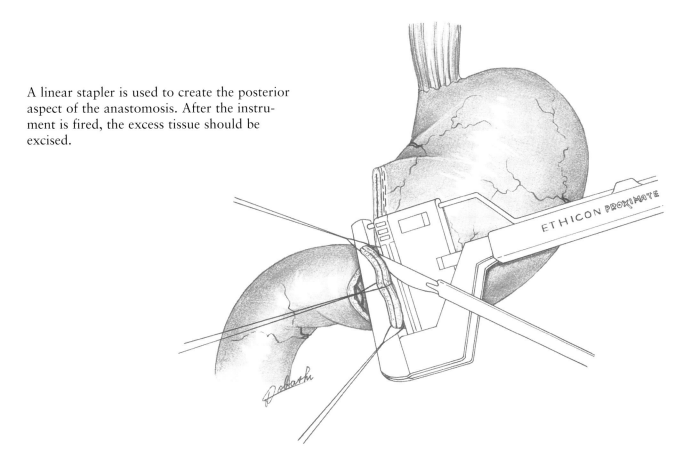

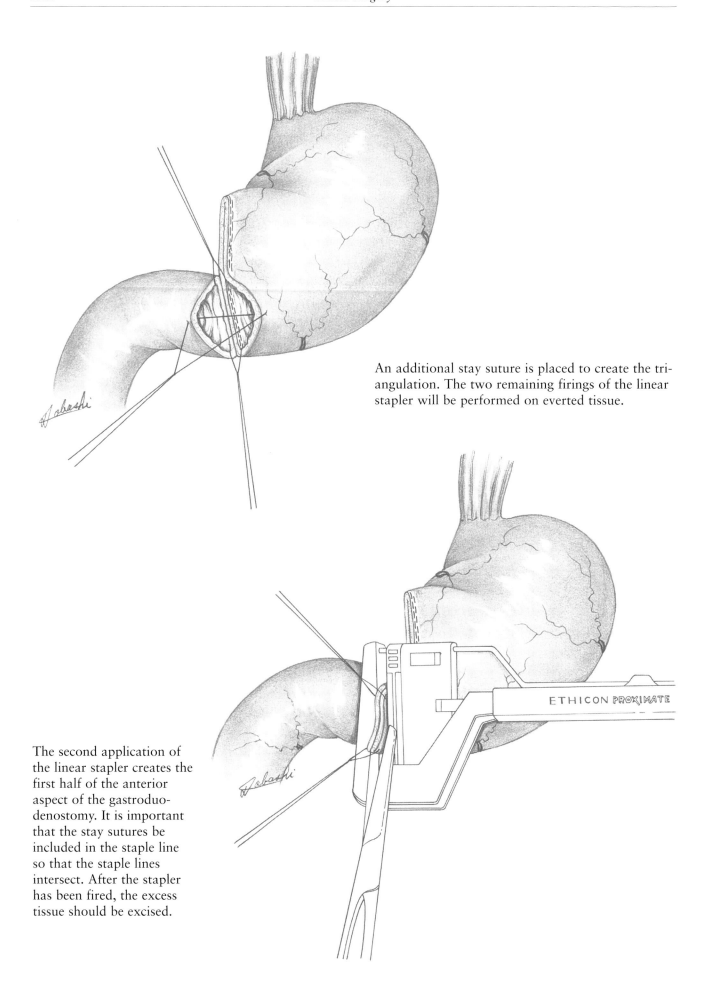

An additional stay suture is placed to create the triangulation. The two remaining firings of the linear stapler will be performed on everted tissue.

The second application of the linear stapler creates the first half of the anterior aspect of the gastroduodenostomy. It is important that the stay sutures be included in the staple line so that the staple lines intersect. After the stapler has been fired, the excess tissue should be excised.

ETHICON PROXIMATE

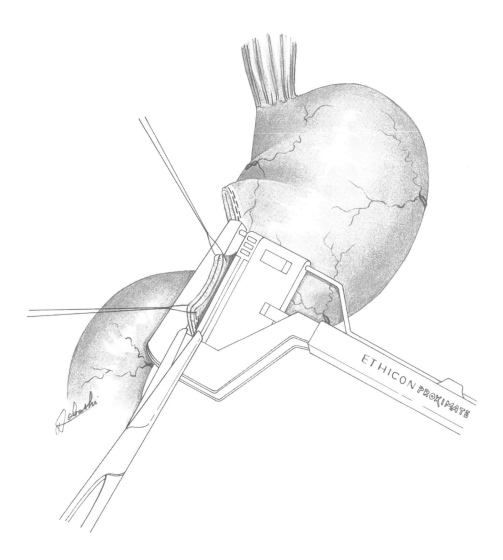

Triangulation is completed with the third firing of the linear stapler, creating the second half of the anterior aspect of the anastomosis. In doing this, the same principles previously described should be adhered to.

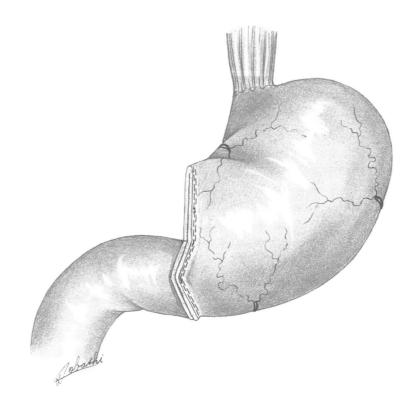

End result.

Billroth II

Subtotal Gastrectomy with a Side-to-Side Gastrojejunostomy (with Circular Stapler)

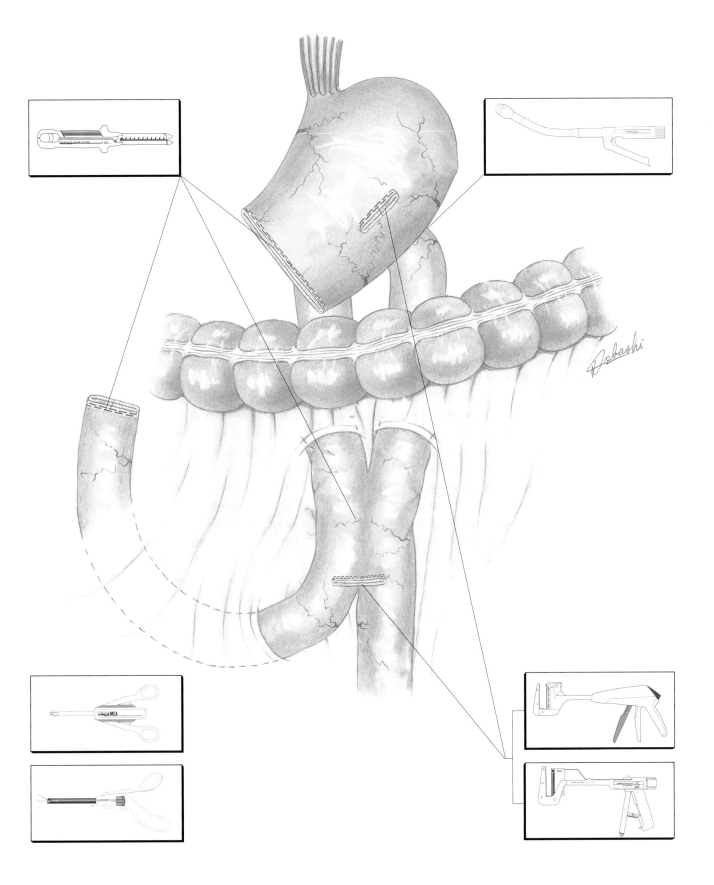

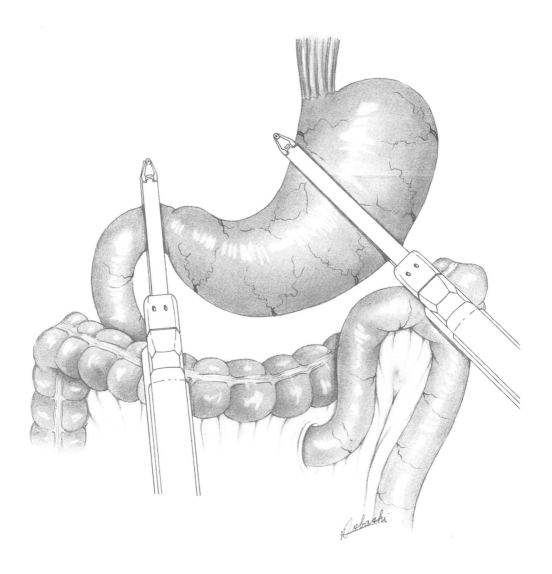

The procedure begins with mobilization of the stomach using suture ligatures, clips, or the Harmonic Scalpel. A subtotal gastrectomy is performed with two firings of the linear cutter. After firing, the staple lines should be examined for hemostasis and proper staple closure.

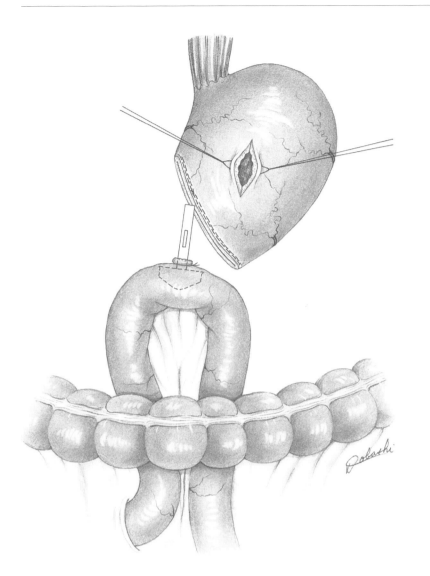

A jejunal loop is brought through the transverse mesocolon and positioned adjacent to the gastric remnant.

A purse-string suture is placed in the antimesenteric border of the jejunum at the site of the proposed anastomosis. A jejunotomy is created in the center of the purse-string. Circular stapler sizers are used to select the appropriate size circular stapler. The anvil of the circular stapler is inserted into the jejunum, and the purse-string suture is tied. The anterior gastric wall is then incised at least 3 cm superior to the staple line in the remaining stomach.

The circular stapler is inserted through the gastrotomy, and the posterior gastric wall is pierced with the trocar at the proposed anastomotic site. This should be at least 3 cm superior to the gastric staple line. The anvil is attached to the integral trocar and the circular stapler is closed and fired, creating the side-to-side gastrojejunostomy. After the circular stapler is withdrawn, the tissue donuts are examined. The donuts should be intact and include all tissue layers. If the donuts are not complete, the anastomosis should be carefully checked for leakage and appropriate repairs made.

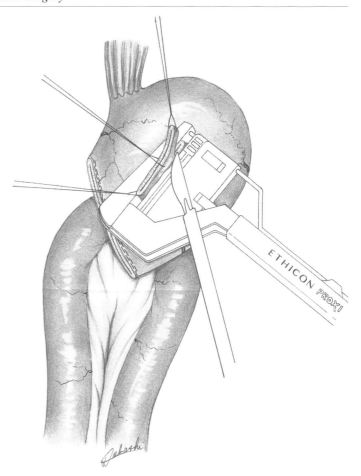

The gastrotomy is closed using a linear stapler, and any excess tissue is excised.

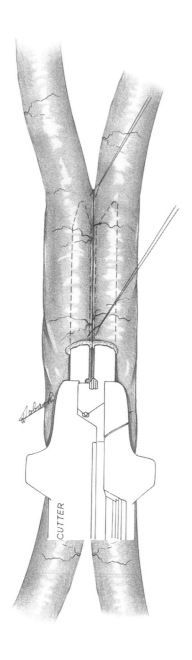

A jejunojejunostomy (Braun technique) is formed by creating enterotomies on the antimesenteric borders of the loops of the jejunum to be anastomosed. The forks of the linear cutter are introduced into the enterotomies, the instrument is closed and fired, and the jejunojejunostomy is created.

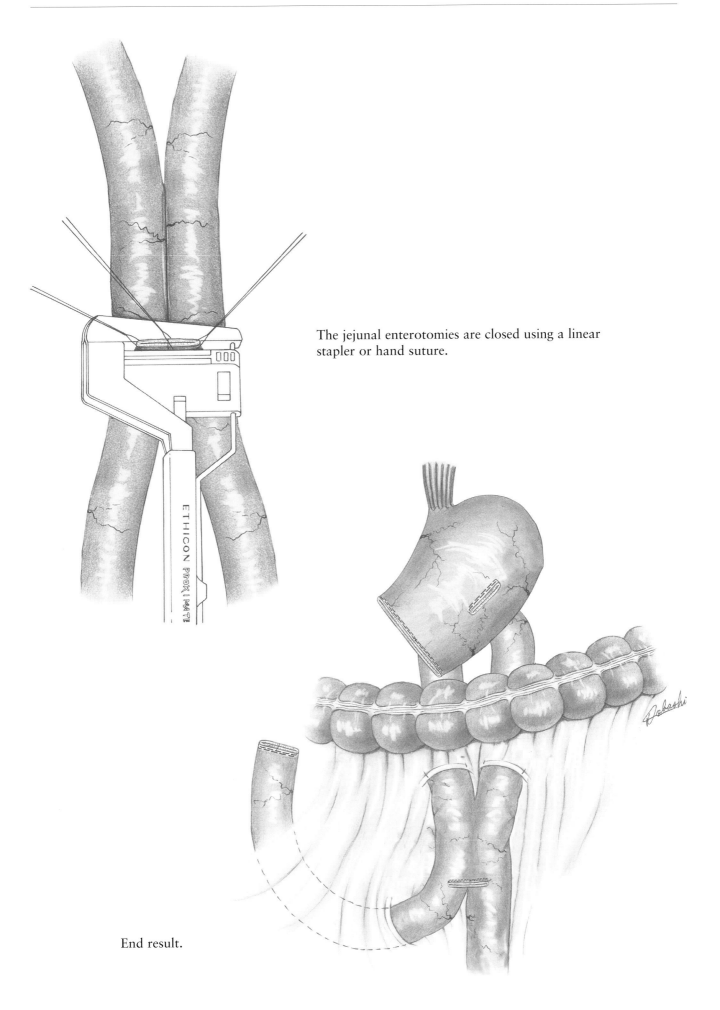

The jejunal enterotomies are closed using a linear stapler or hand suture.

End result.

Billroth II

Subtotal Gastrectomy with a Side-to-Side Gastrojejunostomy (with Linear Cutter)

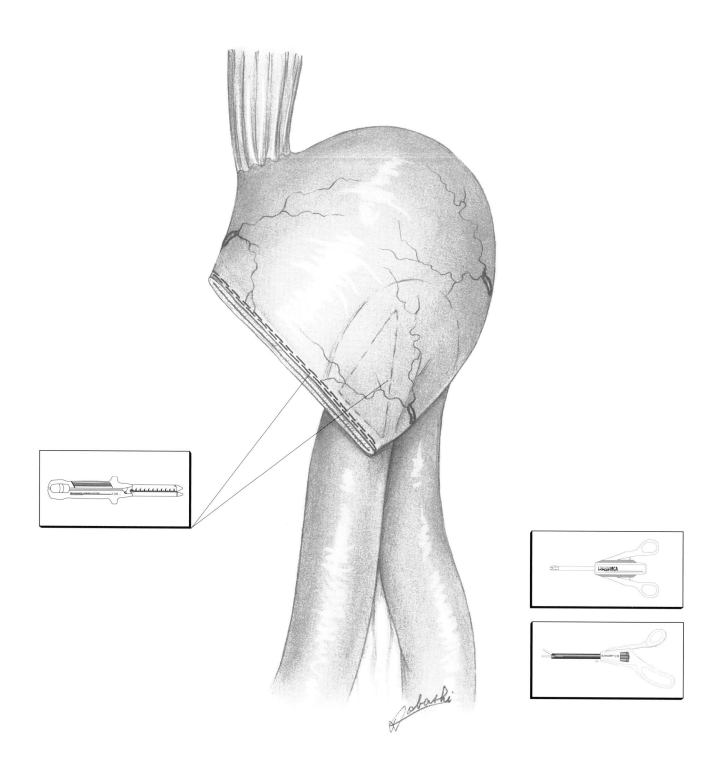

Alternative technique, in which the gastrojejunostomy
is performed with a linear cutter.

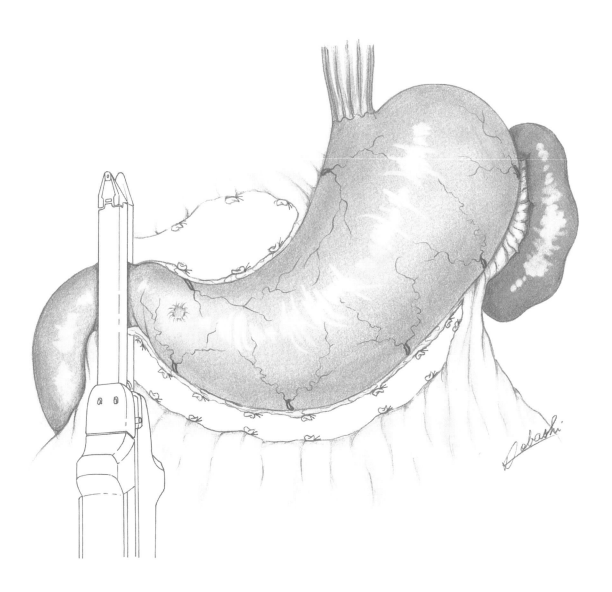

The procedure begins with mobilization of the stomach using suture ligatures, clips, or the Harmonic Scalpel. The duodenum is transected with a linear cutter, and the staple line is examined for hemostasis and proper staple closure.

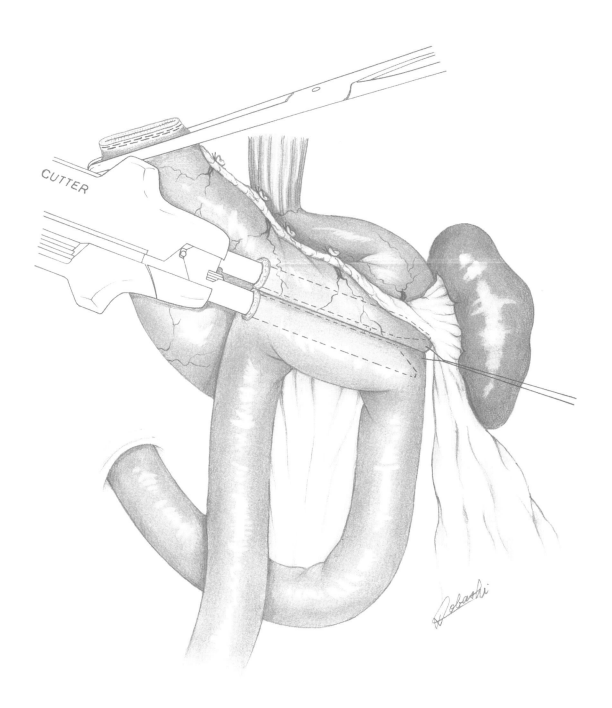

Pulling up a Jejunal Loop

Incisions are made on the antimesenteric border of the jejunum and
the posterior gastric wall approximately 3 cm from the greater
curvature. A side-to-side gastrojejunostomy is created using the
linear cutter. The staple line is examined for hemostasis and proper
staple closure. The gastrojejunostomy should be created parallel to,
and 3 cm from, the greater curvature.

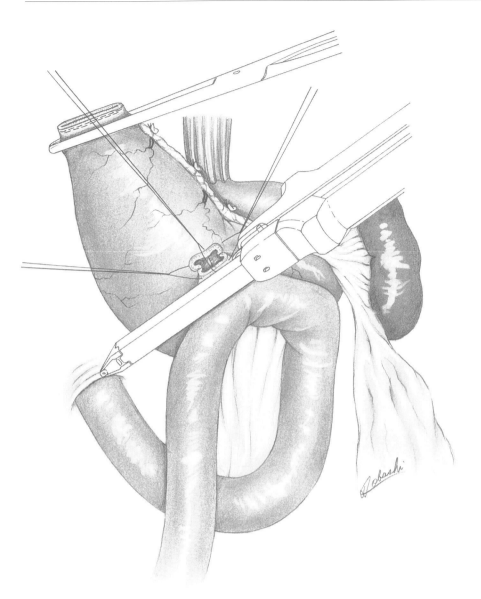

Resection of the stomach and closure of the gastrotomy and jejunal enterotomy are performed simultaneously with a linear cutter. The staple line is then examined for hemostasis and proper closure.

To finish the procedure, a jejunojejunostomy is performed following the Braun technique described previously.

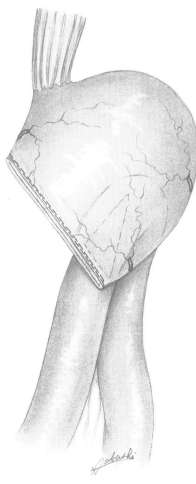

Billroth II (Alternative Technique)

Subtotal Gastrectomy with a Side-to-Side Gastrojejunostomy (with Linear Cutter)

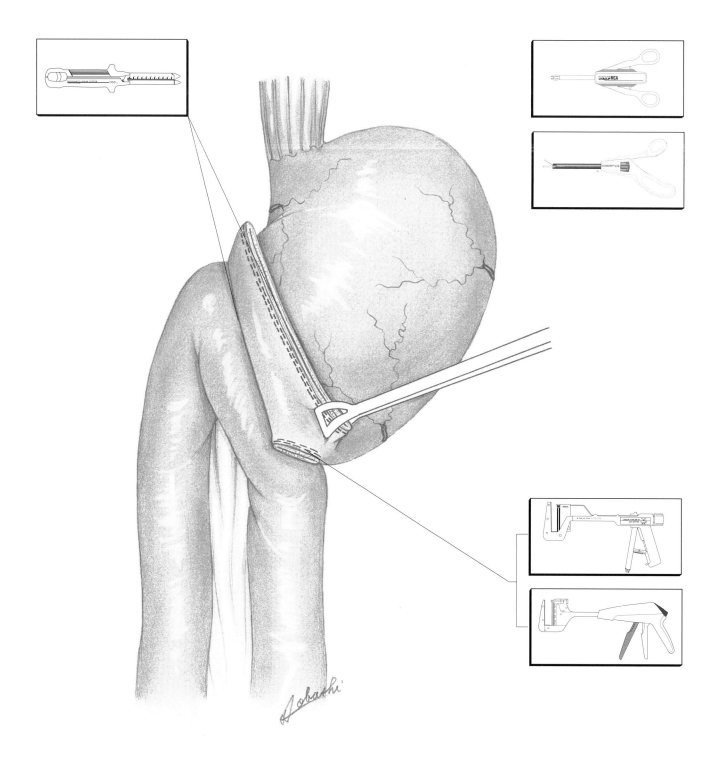

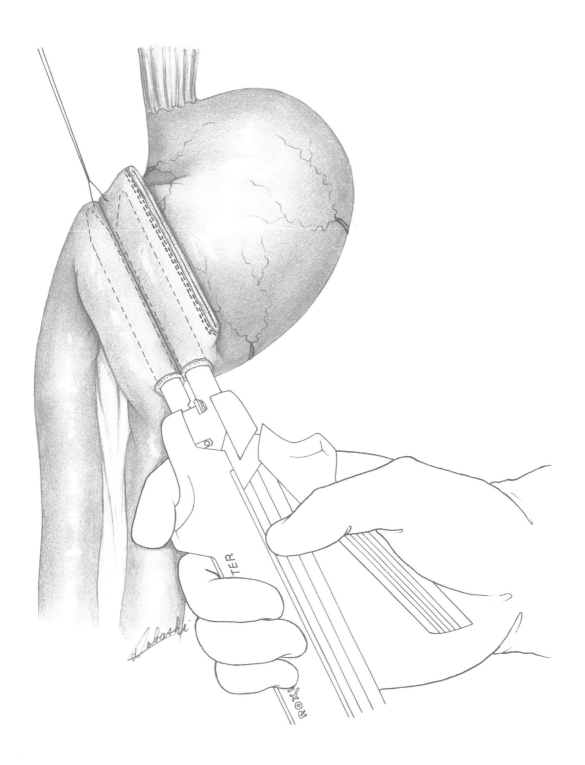

An appropriate loop of jejunum is selected. To introduce the
forks of the linear cutter, incisions are made on the antimesenteric border of the jejunum and on the posterior gastric wall in
the area of the greater curvature approximately 3 cm from the
gastric staple line. A side-to-side gastrojejunostomy is then created using the linear cutter. The gastrojejunostomy should be
parallel to, and 3 cm proximal to, the distal gastric staple line.
The staple lines are examined for hemostasis and proper closure.

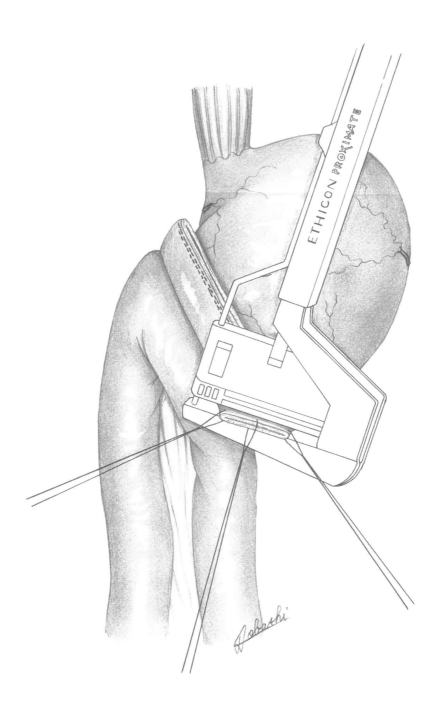

The common opening is closed using a linear stapler.

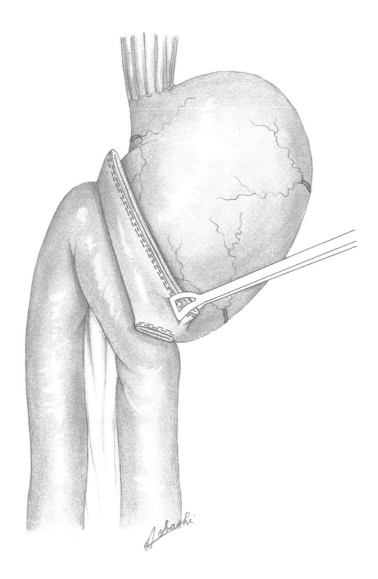

To complete the procedure, a jejunojejunostomy is performed following the Braun technique previously described.

Total Gastrectomy

End-to-Side Jejunal Interposition (Longmire-Gütgemann)

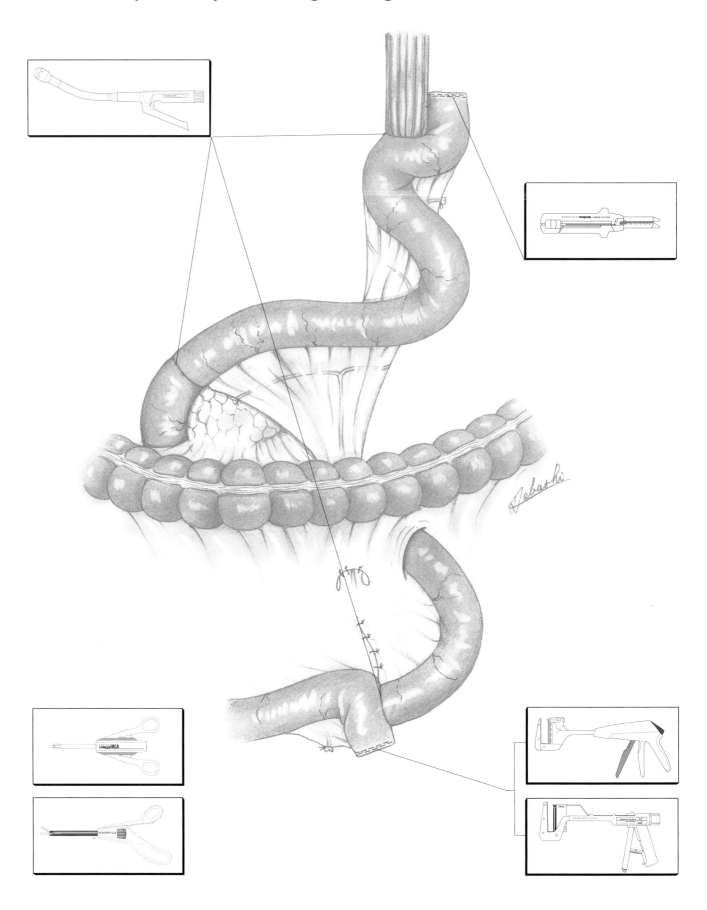

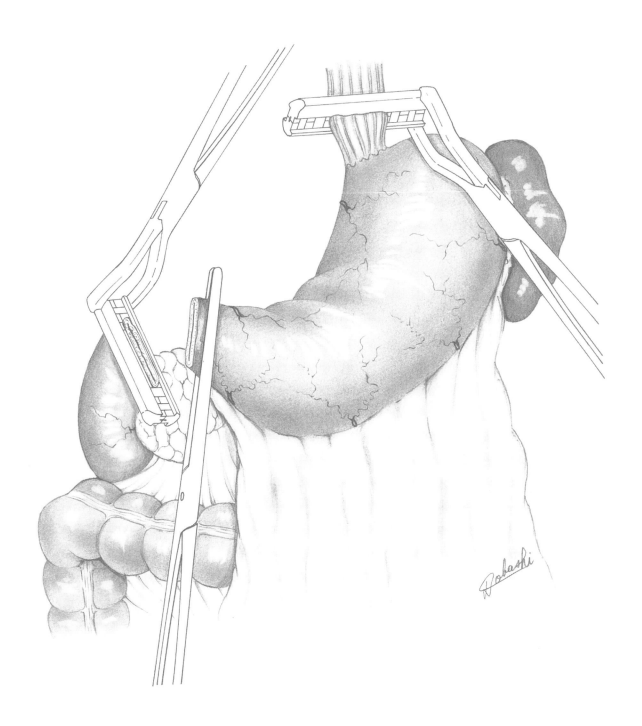

The procedure begins with mobilization of the stomach
using suture ligatures, clips, or the Harmonic Scalpel.
A purse-string suture is placed on the first portion of the
duodenum using a purse-string suture clamp. The distal
line of transection is created by cutting along the guide of
the duodenal purse-string suture clamp. A second purse-
string suture clamp is placed on the distal esophagus.
The specimen can then be completely resected by cutting
along the guide of the esophageal purse-string suture
clamp.

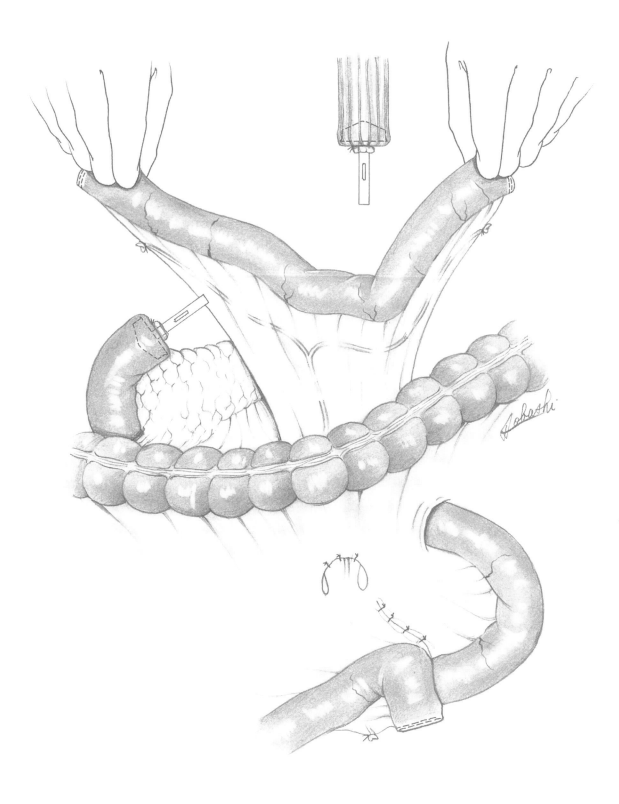

The appropriate circular stapler is determined by using the circular stapler sizers. The anvil of a circular stapler is inserted into the esophagus, and another anvil is inserted into the duodenum. The purse-string sutures are tied to secure the anvils in place. Next, by firing the linear cutter twice, a 50-cm jejunal segment is isolated for use as a gastric replacement. The continuity of the jejunum is reestablished by creating an end-to-side jejunojejunostomy using a circular stapler and a linear stapler. After the circular stapler is withdrawn, the tissue donuts are examined for completeness. The donuts should be intact and include all tissue layers. If the donuts are not complete, the anastomosis should be carefully checked for leakage and appropriate repairs made.

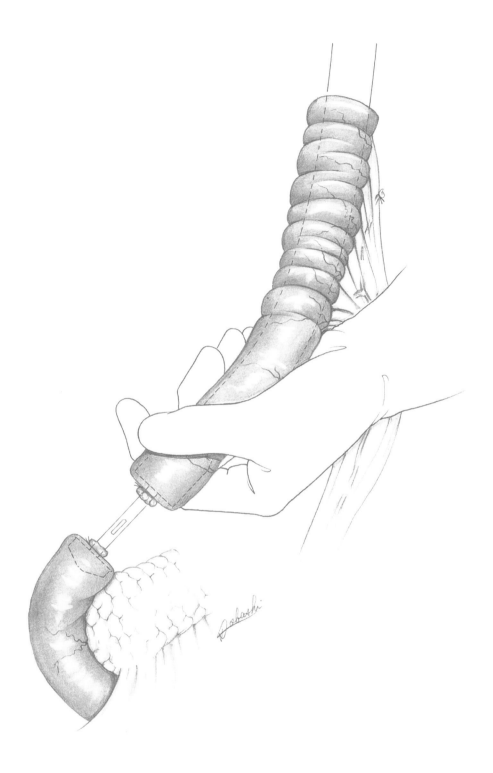

A purse-string suture clamp is placed at the distal end of the jejunal interposition segment, and a purse-string suture is created. A scalpel is used to resect any excess tissue along the cutting guide, including the staple line at the distal end of the interposition segment. After the proximal staple line of the jejunal interposition has been resected, the shaft of the circular stapler is threaded through the interposition segment, and the purse-string suture is tied around the trocar. This step must be performed with extreme care, to avoid injury to the bowel and the possibility of later fistula development. The anvil is attached to the integral trocar, and the stapler is closed and fired, creating the end-to-end jejunoduodenostomy. After the circular stapler is withdrawn, the tissue donuts are examined for completeness. The donuts should be intact and include all tissue layers. If the donuts are not complete, the anastomosis should be carefully checked for leakage and appropriate repairs made.

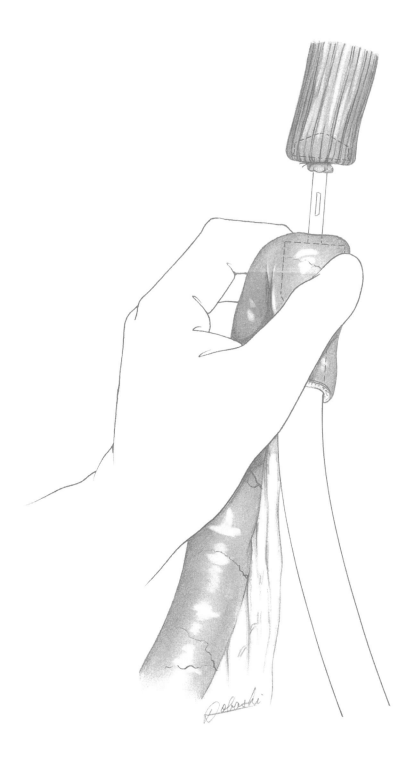

A circular stapler is then inserted into the proximal end of the jejunal interposition segment. The integral trocar is advanced, and the bowel wall is pierced by the trocar on the antimesenteric side of the interposition segment, about 5 cm from the proximal end. The anvil is attached to the integral trocar and the circular stapler is closed and fired, creating the end-to-side esophagojejunostomy. The circular stapler is withdrawn, and the tissue donuts are examined for completeness. The donuts should be intact and include all tissue layers. If the donuts are not complete, the anastomosis should be carefully checked for leakage and appropriate repairs made.

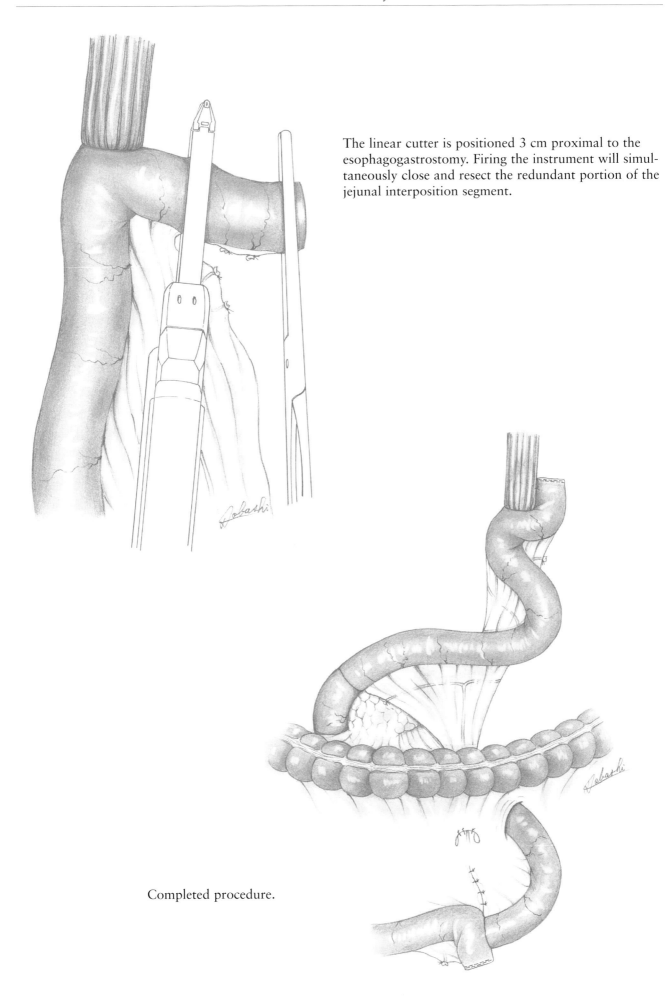

The linear cutter is positioned 3 cm proximal to the esophagogastrostomy. Firing the instrument will simultaneously close and resect the redundant portion of the jejunal interposition segment.

Completed procedure.

Total Gastrectomy

End-to-End Jejunal Interposition (Alternative Technique)

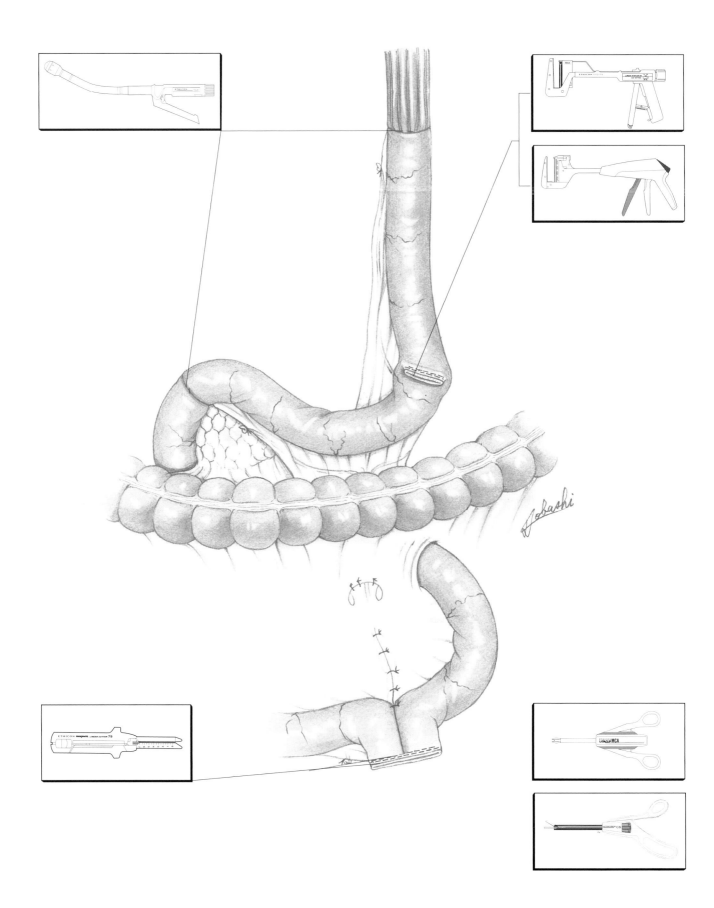

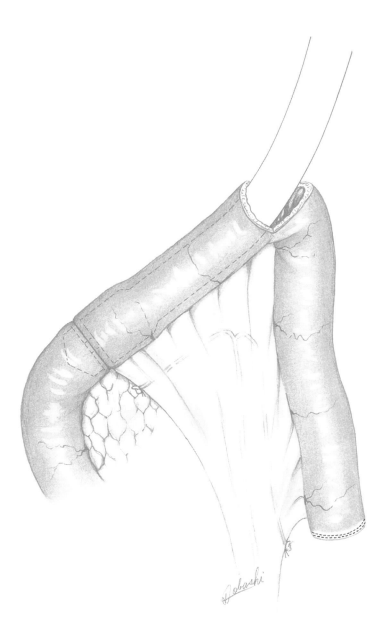

After the total gastrectomy is performed, and an isolated jejunal interposition segment has been prepared, small bowel continuity is reestablished by creating a functional end-to-end anastomosis using a linear cutter. Three purse-string sutures are placed after excising the duodenal, esophageal, and distal jejunal interposition segment staple lines. The anvil of an appropriately sized circular stapler is inserted into the lumens of both the duodenum and esophagus, and the corresponding purse-string sutures are tied around the anvils' center rods. A transverse enterotomy is made in the jejunal interposition segment. The shaft of the appropriate circular stapler is introduced through the jejunal enterotomy and passed to the distal end of the interposition segment. The previously placed purse-string suture is tied around the integral trocar of the circular stapler. The anvil in the duodenum is attached to the integral trocar, and the circular stapler is closed and fired, creating the end-to-end jejunoduodenostomy. After the circular stapler is withdrawn, the tissue donuts are examined for completeness. The donuts should be intact and include all tissue layers. If the donuts are not complete, the anastomosis should be carefully checked for leakage and appropriate repairs made.

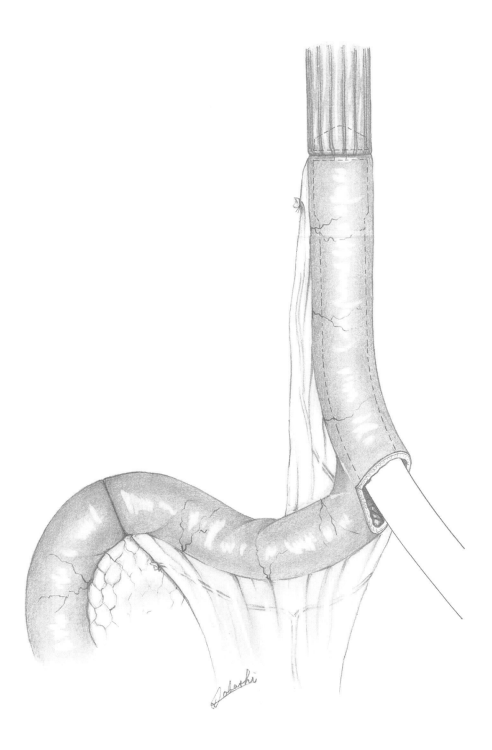

After the staple line is resected at the proximal end of the jejunal interposition segment, a purse-string suture is placed at the proximal end of the segment. A second circular stapler is introduced into the jejunal inter-position segment through the enterotomy and passed to the proximal end of the segment. The purse-string suture at the proximal end of the segment is tied around the integral trocar. The esophageal anvil is attached to the integral trocar, and the circular stapler is closed and fired, creating the end-to-end esophago-jejunostomy. After the circular stapler is withdrawn, the tissue donuts are examined for completeness. The tissue donuts should be intact and include all tissue layers. If the donuts are not complete, the ana-stomosis should be carefully checked for leakage and appropriate repairs made.

Note: The preferred hand-sewn technique for a purse-string suture at the esophagus is the whip stitch.

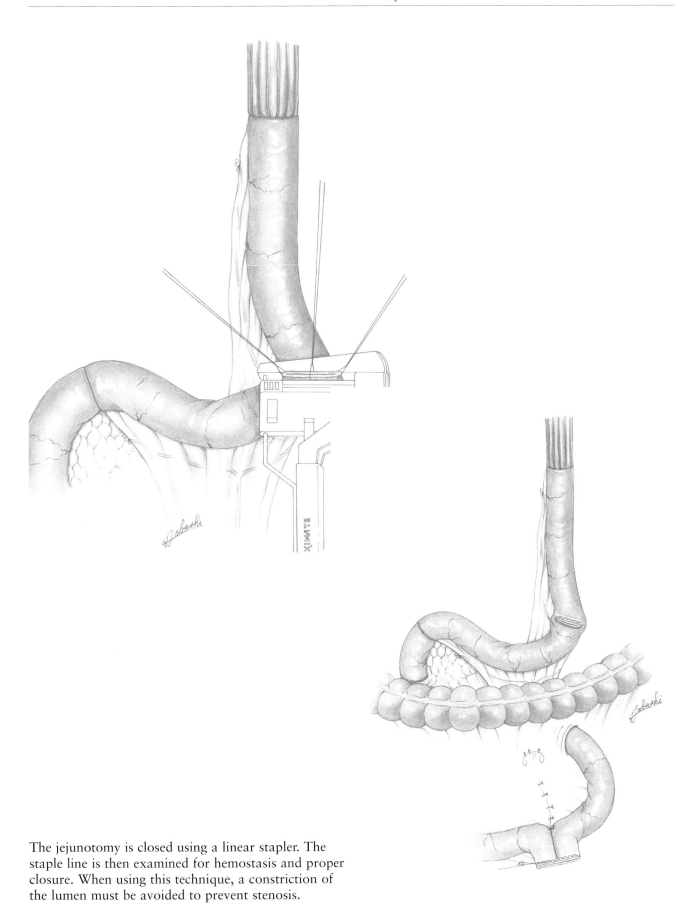

The jejunotomy is closed using a linear stapler. The staple line is then examined for hemostasis and proper closure. When using this technique, a constriction of the lumen must be avoided to prevent stenosis.

Total Gastrectomy

Esophagojejunostomy with End-to-Side Roux-en-Y

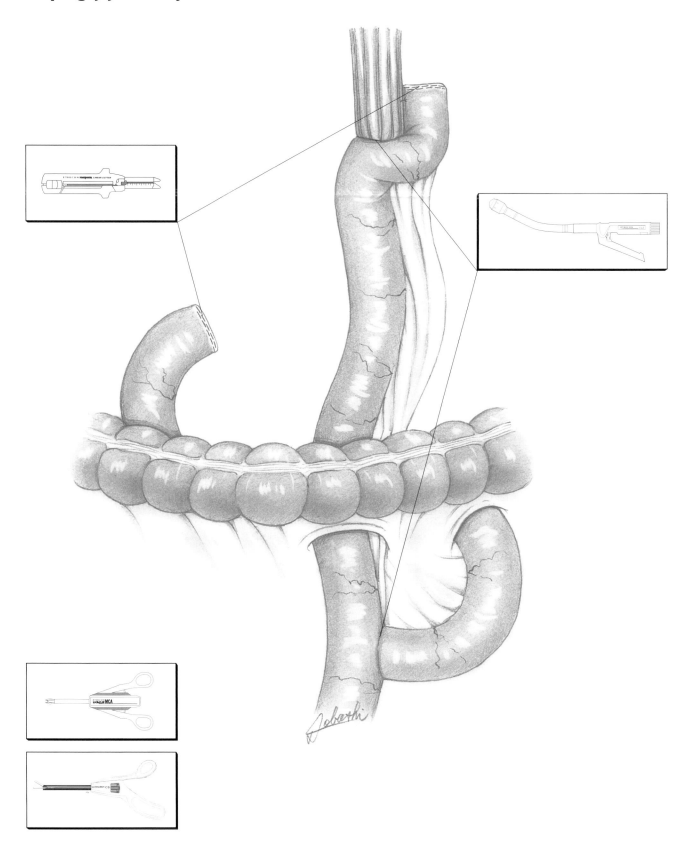

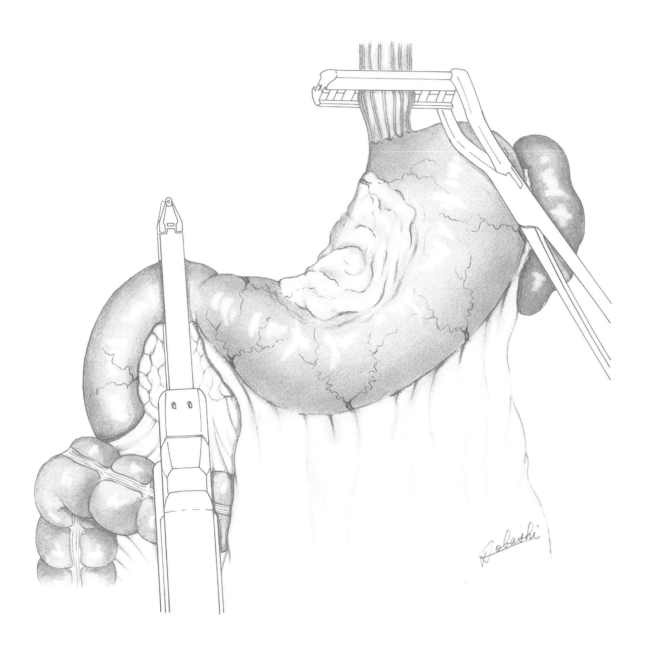

The procedure begins with complete mobilization of the stomach using suture ligatures, clips, or the Harmonic Scalpel. A linear cutter is used to transect the first part of the duodenum and to create the distal line of transection. The staple line is examined for hemostasis and proper closure. A purse-string suture clamp is used to place a purse-string suture on the distal portion of the esophagus. The esophagus is transected along the cutting guide of the purse-string suture clamp. The specimen containing the diseased segment is then removed. Note: If a purse-string suture clamp is not used, the purse-string technique recommended in the esophagus is the whip stitch.

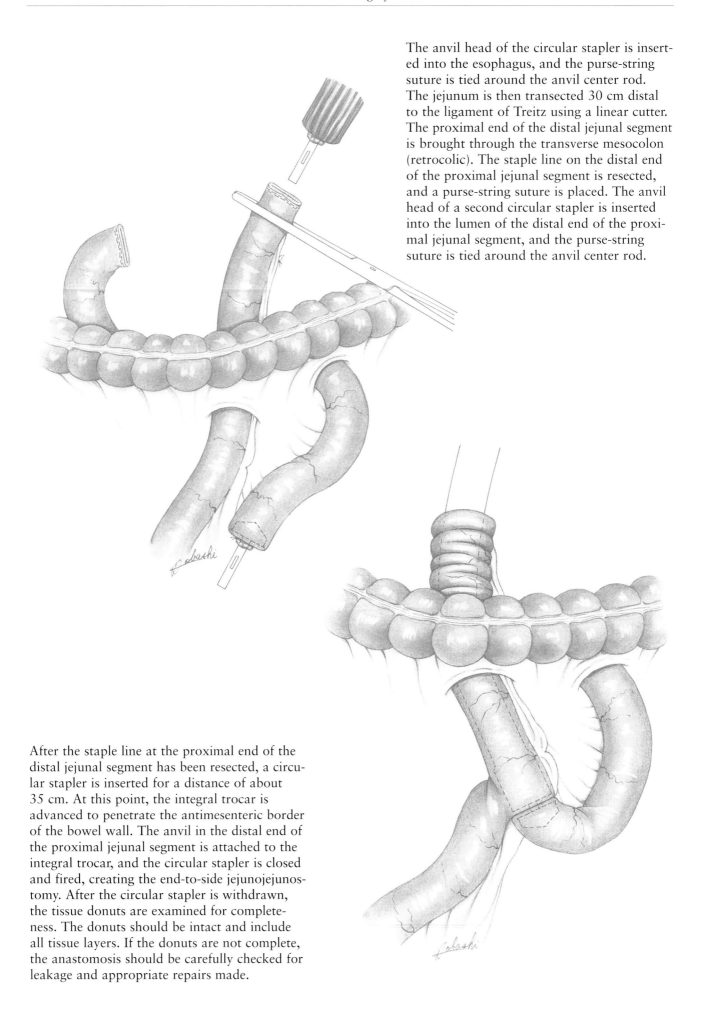

The anvil head of the circular stapler is inserted into the esophagus, and the purse-string suture is tied around the anvil center rod. The jejunum is then transected 30 cm distal to the ligament of Treitz using a linear cutter. The proximal end of the distal jejunal segment is brought through the transverse mesocolon (retrocolic). The staple line on the distal end of the proximal jejunal segment is resected, and a purse-string suture is placed. The anvil head of a second circular stapler is inserted into the lumen of the distal end of the proximal jejunal segment, and the purse-string suture is tied around the anvil center rod.

After the staple line at the proximal end of the distal jejunal segment has been resected, a circular stapler is inserted for a distance of about 35 cm. At this point, the integral trocar is advanced to penetrate the antimesenteric border of the bowel wall. The anvil in the distal end of the proximal jejunal segment is attached to the integral trocar, and the circular stapler is closed and fired, creating the end-to-side jejunojejunostomy. After the circular stapler is withdrawn, the tissue donuts are examined for completeness. The donuts should be intact and include all tissue layers. If the donuts are not complete, the anastomosis should be carefully checked for leakage and appropriate repairs made.

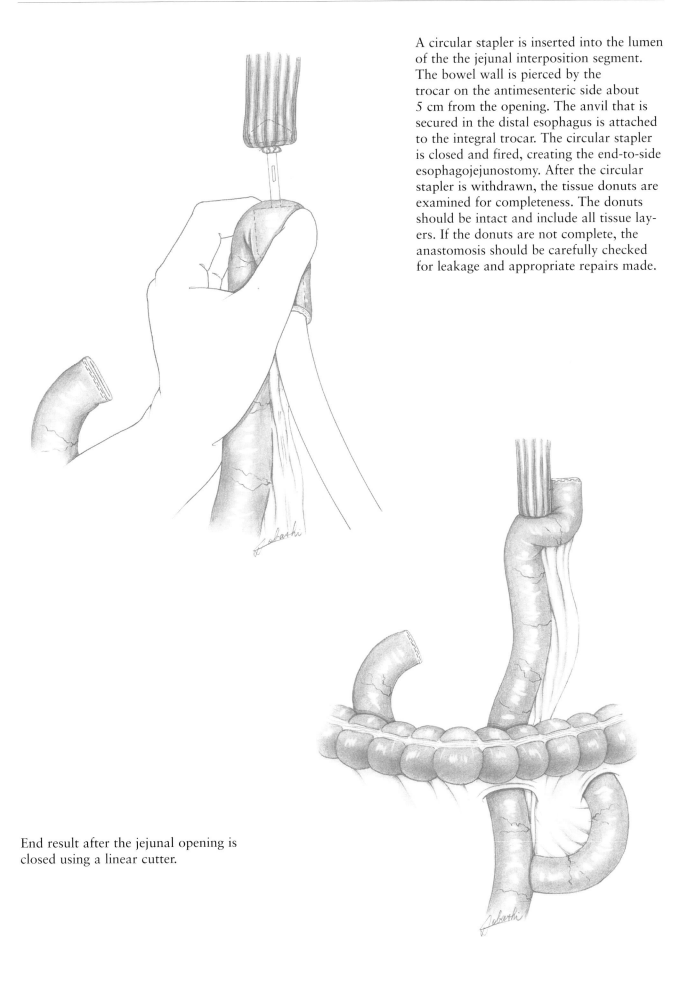

A circular stapler is inserted into the lumen of the the jejunal interposition segment. The bowel wall is pierced by the trocar on the antimesenteric side about 5 cm from the opening. The anvil that is secured in the distal esophagus is attached to the integral trocar. The circular stapler is closed and fired, creating the end-to-side esophagojejunostomy. After the circular stapler is withdrawn, the tissue donuts are examined for completeness. The donuts should be intact and include all tissue layers. If the donuts are not complete, the anastomosis should be carefully checked for leakage and appropriate repairs made.

End result after the jejunal opening is closed using a linear cutter.

Total Gastrectomy

Esophagojejunostomy with a Side-to-Side Roux-en-Y

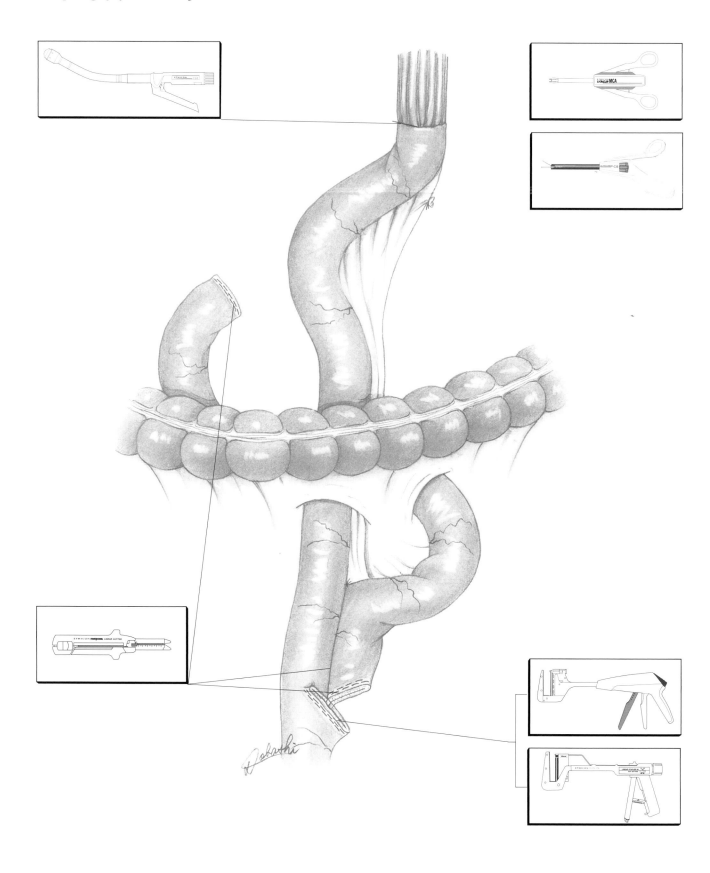

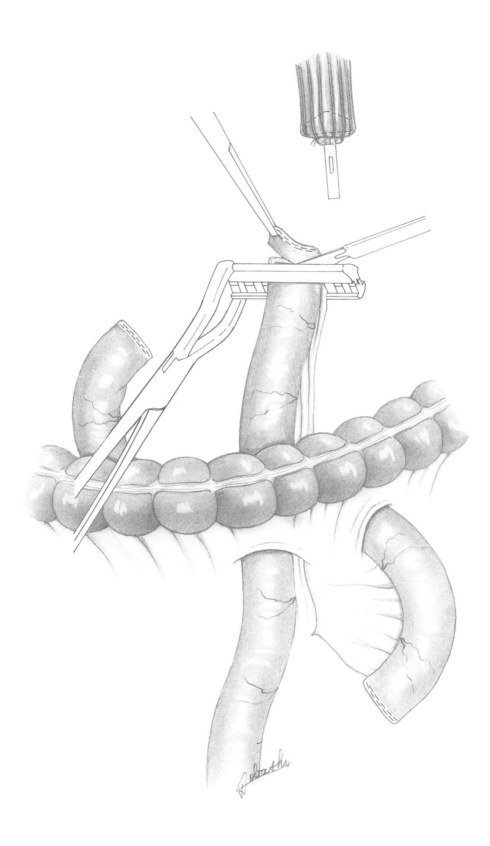

Total gastrectomy and transection of the jejunum are carried out following the steps previously described. The proximal end of the distal jejunal segment is brought to the esophagus in a retrocolic fashion.

The staple line at the proximal end of the distal jejunal segment is resected, and a purse-string suture is placed.

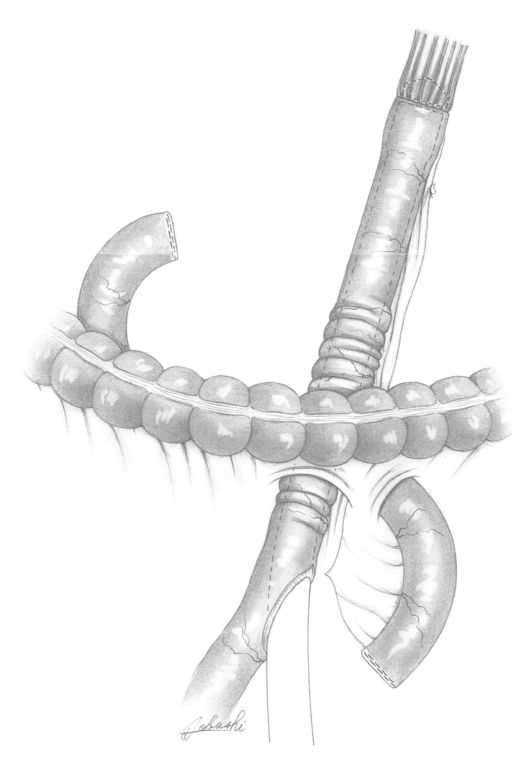

An incision is made on the antimesenteric border of the distal jejunal segment. This incision should be placed 40 cm distal to the proximal end of the distal jejunal segment. The shaft of the appropriate circular stapler is inserted into this jejunotomy and passed to the proximal end of the distal jejunal segment. Extreme care must be taken to avoid damage to the bowel by the stapler. The purse-string suture at the proximal end of the distal jejunal segment is tied around the integral trocar of the stapler.

The anvil that is secured in the lumen of the distal esophagus is attached to the integral trocar, and the circular stapler is closed and fired, creating the end-to-end esophagojejunostomy. After the circular stapler is withdrawn, the tissue donuts are examined for completeness. The donuts should be intact and include all tissue layers. If the donuts are not complete, the anastomosis should be carefully checked for leakage and appropriate repairs made.

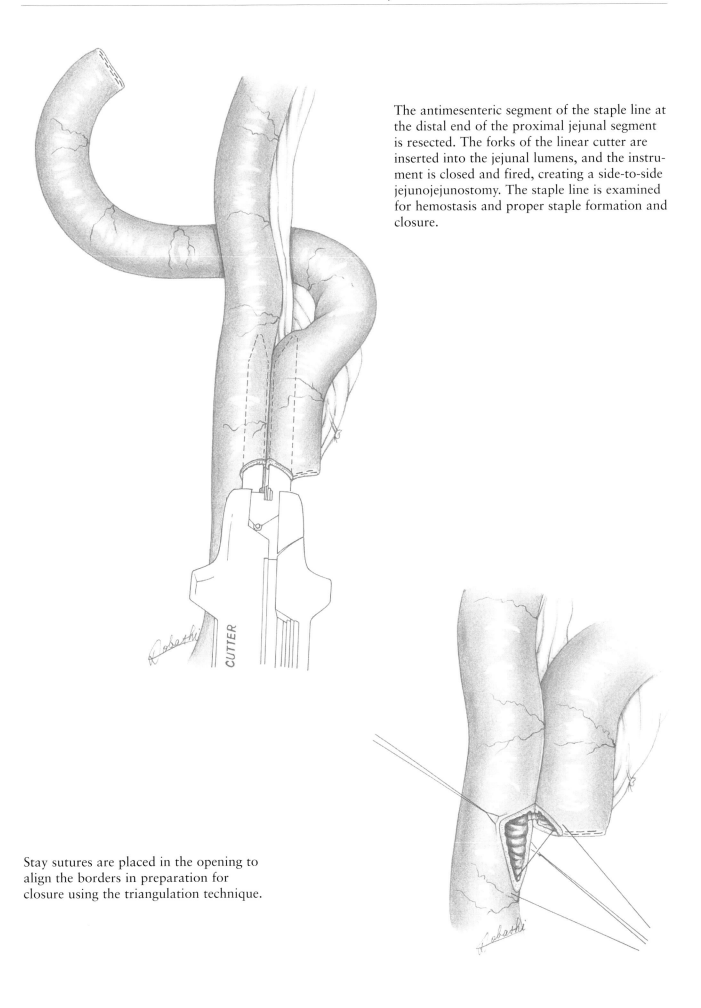

The antimesenteric segment of the staple line at the distal end of the proximal jejunal segment is resected. The forks of the linear cutter are inserted into the jejunal lumens, and the instrument is closed and fired, creating a side-to-side jejunojejunostomy. The staple line is examined for hemostasis and proper staple formation and closure.

Stay sutures are placed in the opening to align the borders in preparation for closure using the triangulation technique.

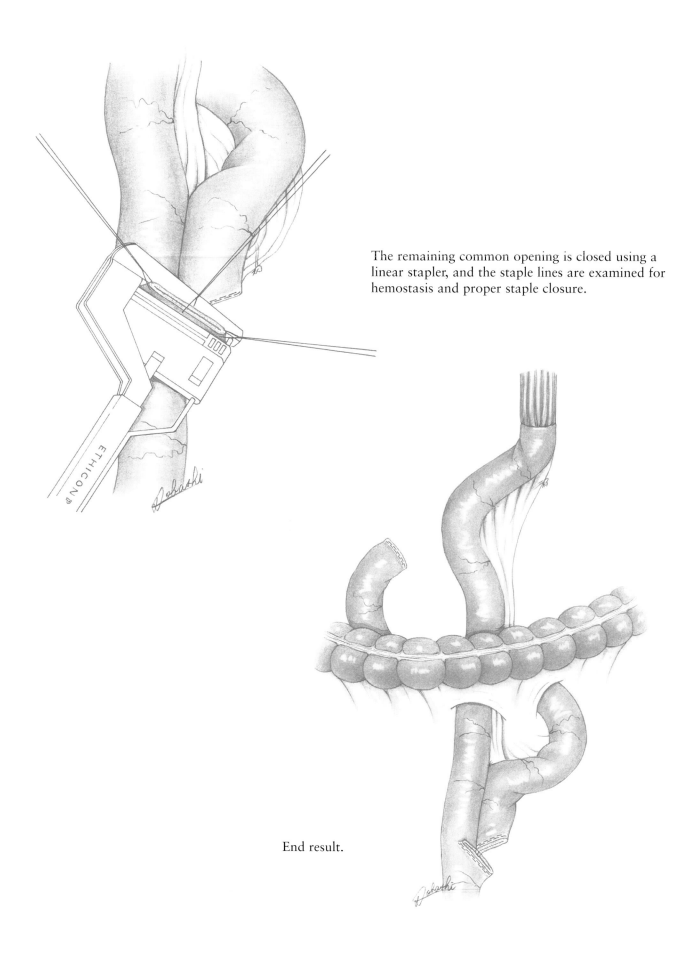

The remaining common opening is closed using a linear stapler, and the staple lines are examined for hemostasis and proper staple closure.

End result.

Total Gastrectomy

Jejunal Interposition with Jejunal Pouch

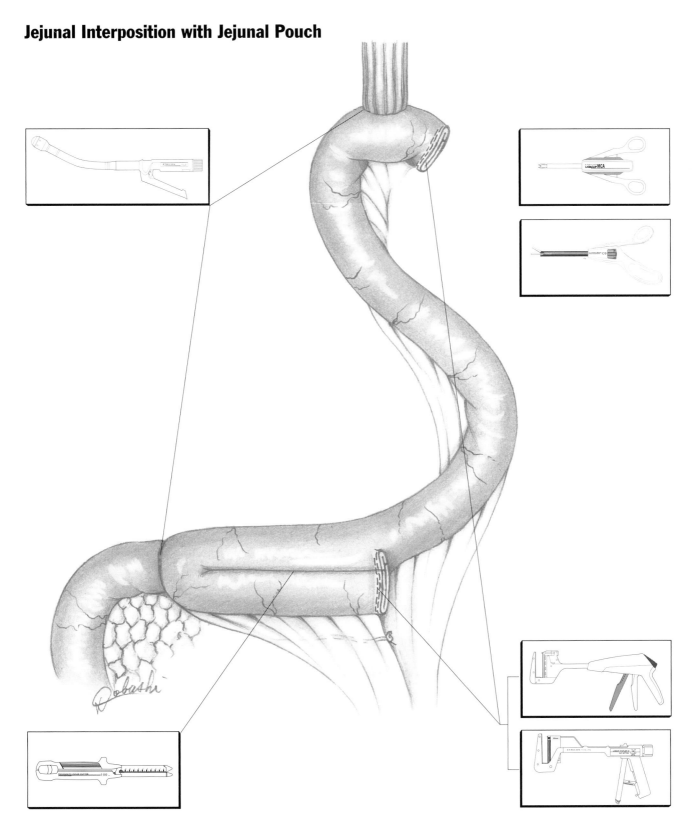

A total gastrectomy and preparation of an isolated jejunal segment are performed as previously described. It is important to ensure that the interposition segment is long enough (55–60 cm) to create the jejunal pouch at the distal end of the interposition segment. An esophagojejunostomy is performed as previously described.

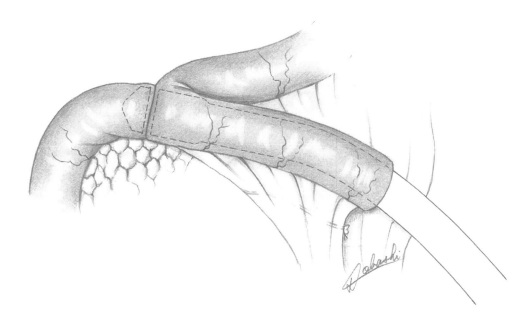

A purse-string suture is placed at the proximal end of the duodenum. The anvil of the circular stapler is inserted into the duodenal lumen, and the purse-string suture is tied around the anvil center rod. The circular stapler is inserted into the lumen of the distal end of the jejunal interposition segment and advanced 10–15 cm. At this point the integral trocar is advanced to pierce the bowel wall on its antimesen- teric border. The anvil is attached to the integral tro- car, and the circular stapler is closed and fired, creat- ing the side-to-end jejunoduodenostomy. After the circular stapler is withdrawn, the tissue donuts are examined for completeness. The donuts should be intact and include all tissue layers. If the donuts are not complete, the anastomosis should be carefully checked for leakage and appropriate repairs made.

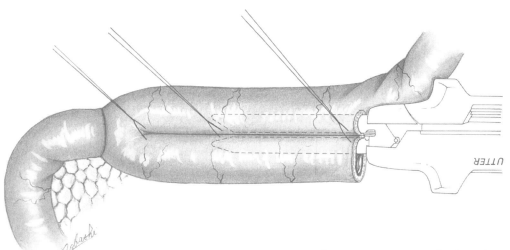

Stay sutures are applied to align the antimesenteric borders of the jejunum that will form the pouch. An enterotomy is performed in order to insert the forks of the linear cutter. The instrument is inserted, closed, and fired, constructing the first anastomotic tract. If the length of the linear cutter is sufficiently long, this step can be carried out with only one firing.

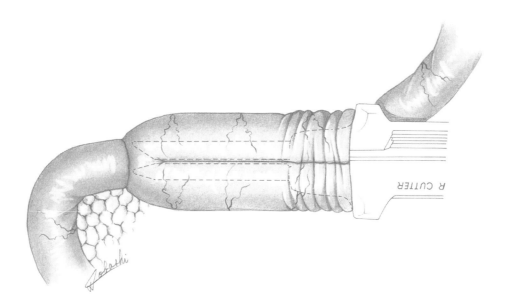

If a second firing is needed to complete the pouch, the anastomosed bowel can be telescoped over the instrument in order to render its distal part accessible.

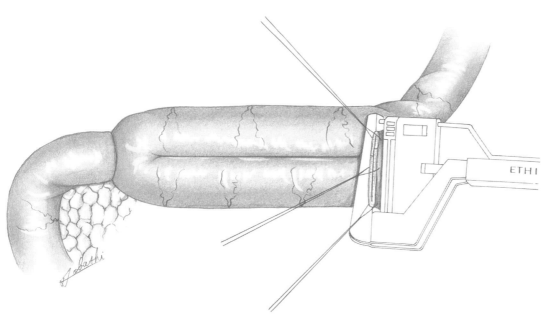

The common opening is closed using a linear stapler aided by stay sutures.

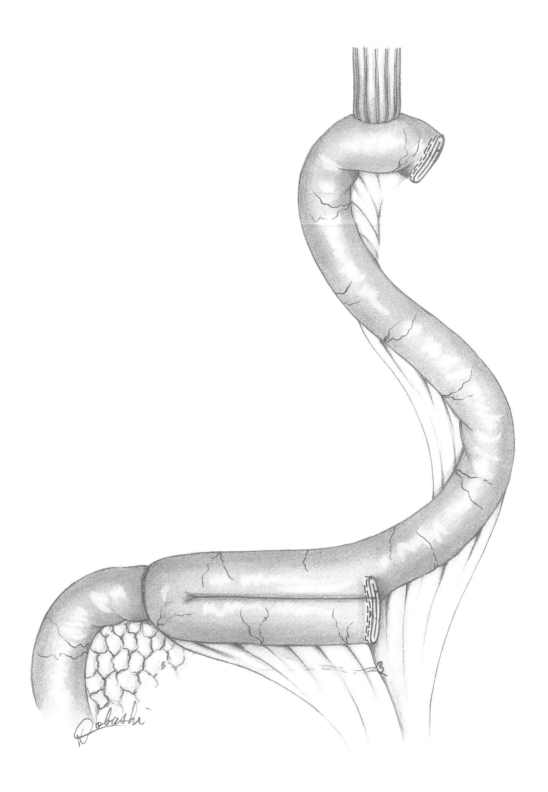

End result.

Total Gastrectomy

Paulino Pouch

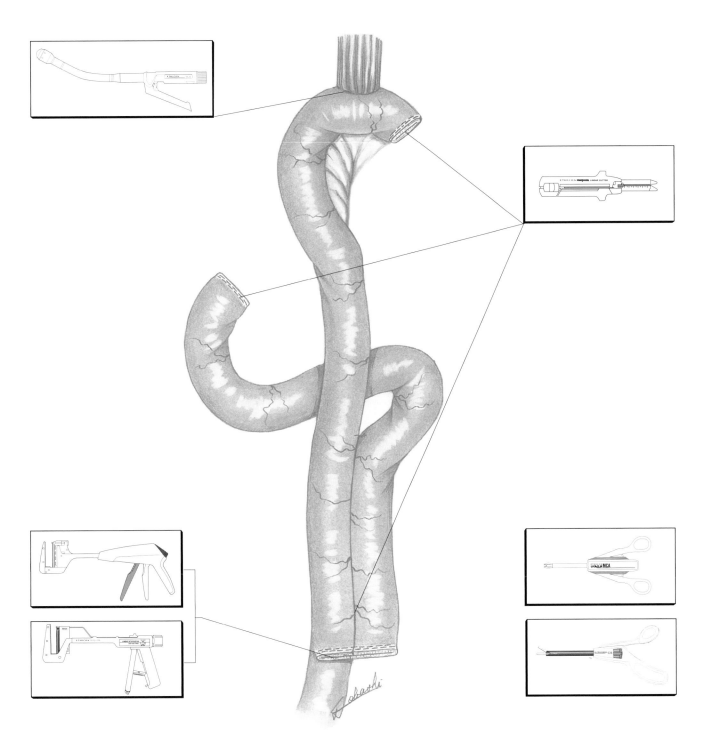

A total gastrectomy is performed. The jejunum is then transected 40–45 cm distal to the ligament of Treitz. An esophagojejunostomy is performed as previously described.

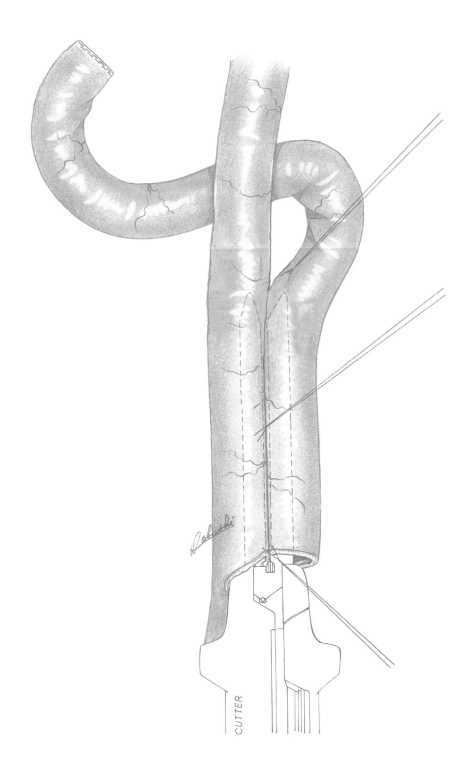

The staple line from the distal end of the proximal jejunal segment is excised. Stay sutures are applied to align the antimesenteric borders of the two portions of the jejunum. An enterotomy is created in the distal jejunal segment adjacent to the distal end of the proximal jejunal segment. The jaws of the linear cutter are inserted, closed, and fired, constructing the first anastomotic tract. If the linear cutter is sufficiently long, this step can be done with only one firing.

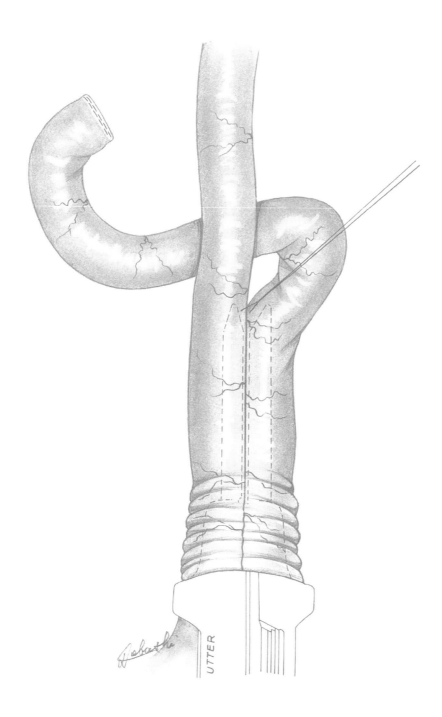

When a second firing is needed to complete the
pouch, the anastomosed bowel can be telescoped
over the instrument in order to render its distal part
accessible.

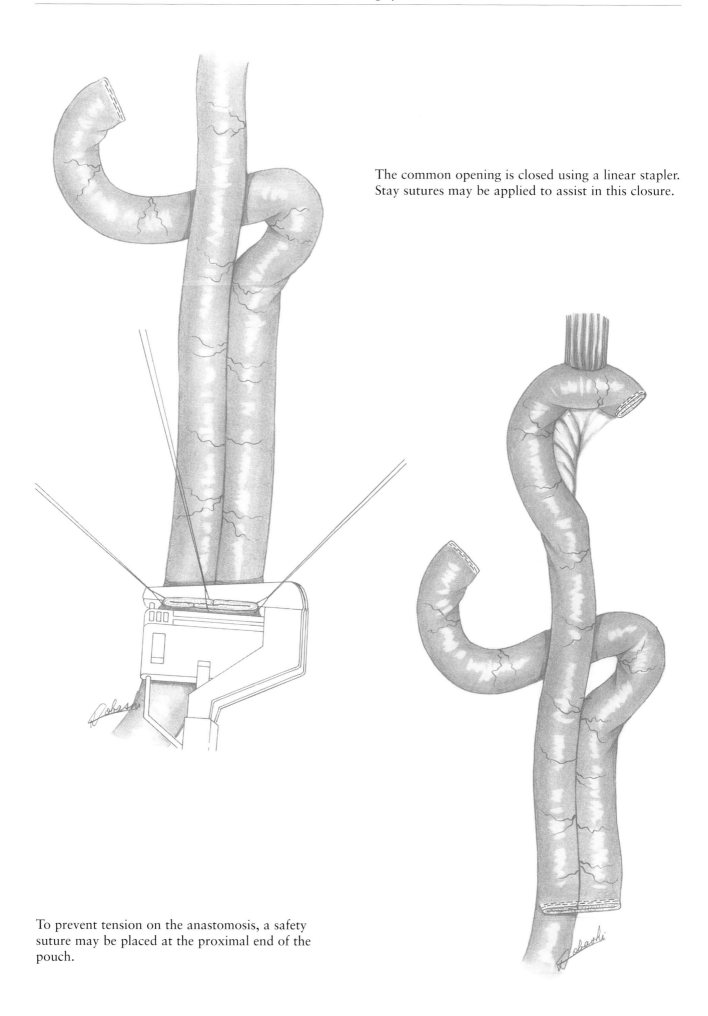

The common opening is closed using a linear stapler. Stay sutures may be applied to assist in this closure.

To prevent tension on the anastomosis, a safety suture may be placed at the proximal end of the pouch.

Total Gastrectomy

Hunt-Lawrence Pouch

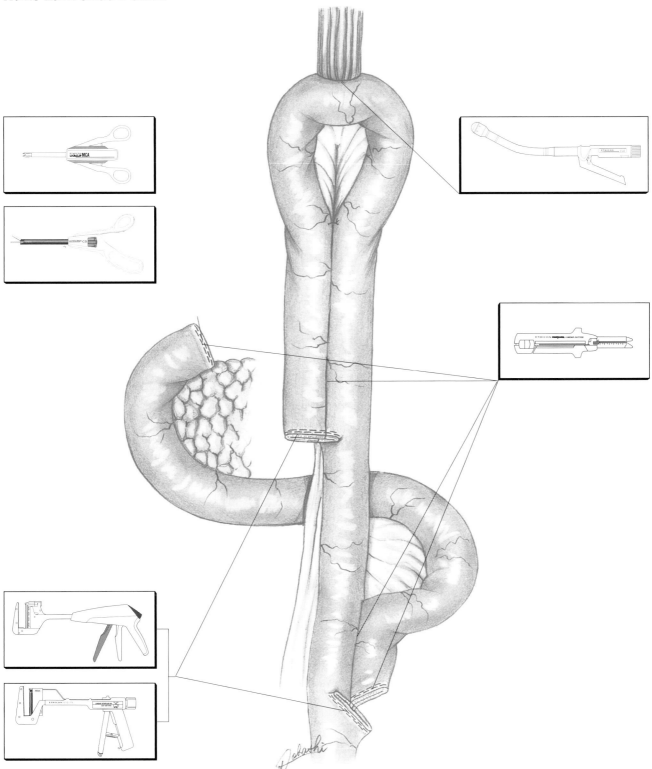

In this procedure the following steps are performed as previously described:
– A total gastrectomy
– Transection of the jejunum 30 cm distal to the ligament of Treitz
– A side-to-side jejunojejunostomy (Roux-en-Y) 60–65 cm distal to the
  proximal end of the distal jejunal segment

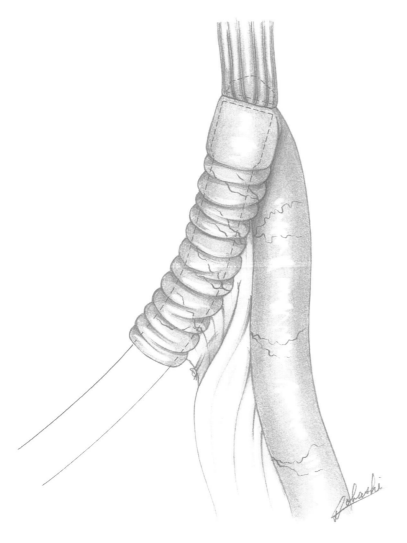

Following placement of a purse-string suture on the distal end of esophagus, the anvil of the circular stapler is inserted into the esophageal lumen, and the purse-string suture is tied around the anvil's center rod. The circular stapler is inserted into the lumen of the proximal end of the distal segment of the jejunum and advanced 25 cm. At this point the bowel wall is pierced by the integral trocar on its antimesenteric border. The anvil is attached to the integral trocar, and the circular stapler is closed and fired, creating the end-to-side esophagojejunostomy. After the circular stapler is withdrawn, the tissue donuts are examined for completeness. The donuts should be intact and include all tissue layers. If the donuts are not complete, the anastomosis should be carefully checked for leakage and appropriate repairs made.

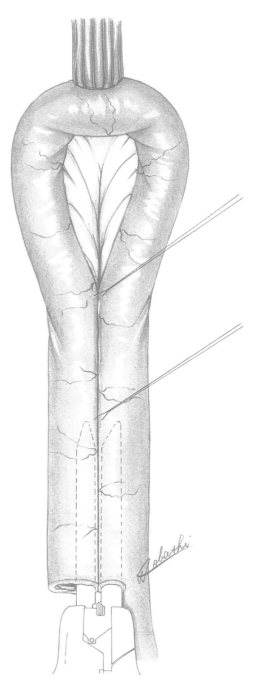

Stay sutures are placed to align the antimesenteric borders of the two portions of the jejunum that will form the pouch. A jejunotomy is created in the segment of the jejunum adjacent to the open proximal end of the distal jejunal segment. The jaws of the linear cutter are introduced into the jejunal lumens. The instrument is closed and fired, creating the first anastomotic tract.

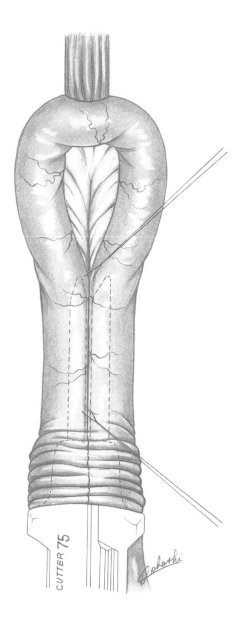

A second firing is needed to complete the pouch. The anastomosed bowel can be telescoped over the instrument in order to render its distal part accessible.

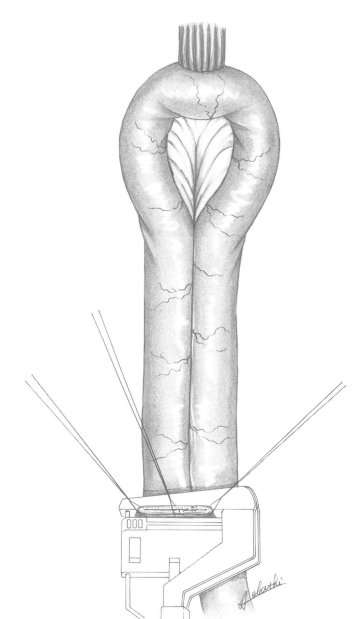

The common opening is closed using a linear stapler. Stay sutures may be used to assist in aligning the tissue edges.

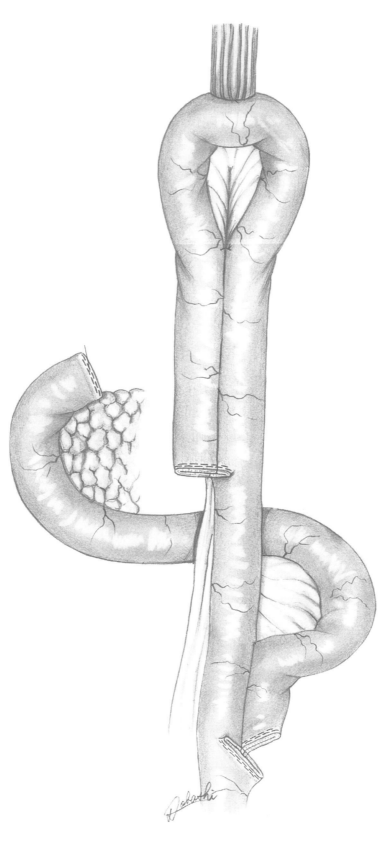

To prevent tension on the anastomosis, a
safety suture is placed at the proximal end of
the pouch.

Pyloroplasty

Heineke-Mikulicz Technique

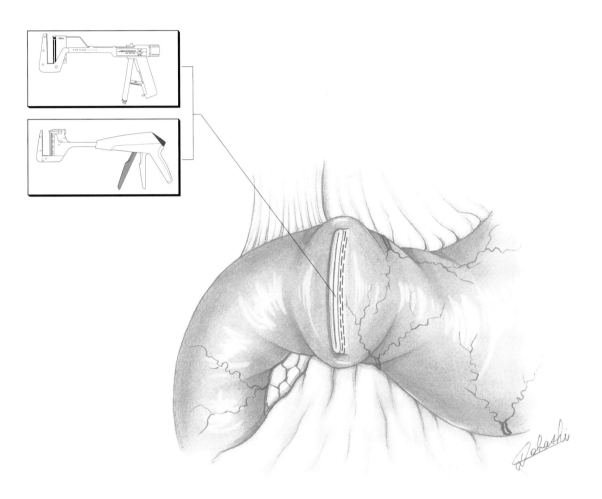

A 3–5-cm transmural incision is made on the anterior aspect of the gastroduodenal junction. It should include the pyloric sphincter and the most proximal portion of the duodenum.

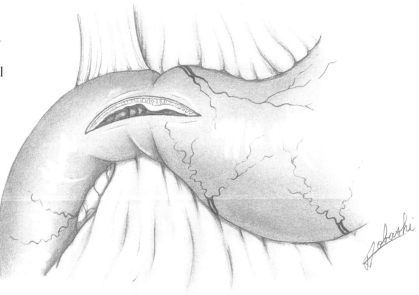

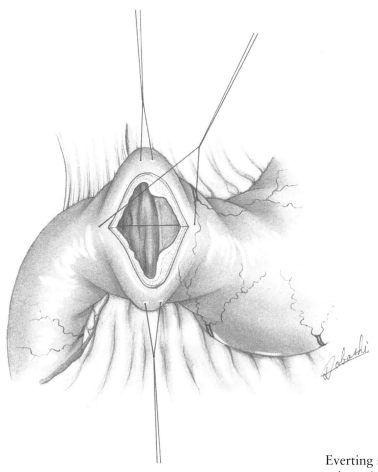

Everting stay sutures are placed to change the orientation of the wound edges from longitudinal to transverse.

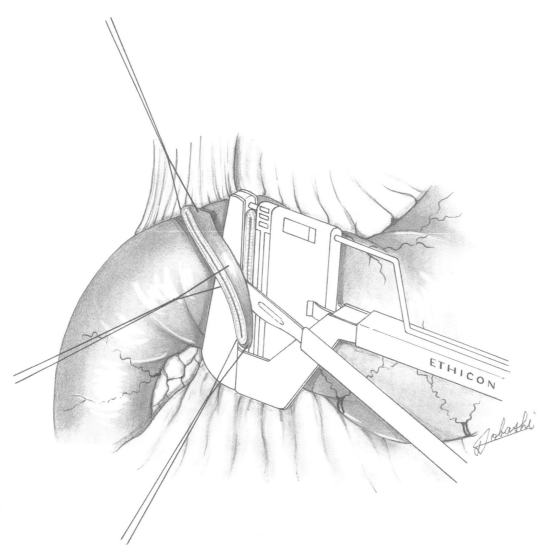

The gastroduodenotomy is closed using a linear stapler, and excess tissue is resected using the cutting edge of the linear stapler as a guide. The staple lines are examined for hemostasis and proper closure.

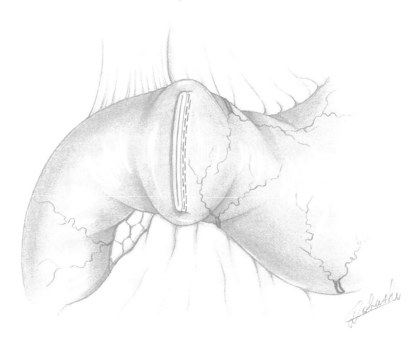

Completed pyloroplasty.

Pyloroplasty

Jaboulay Technique I

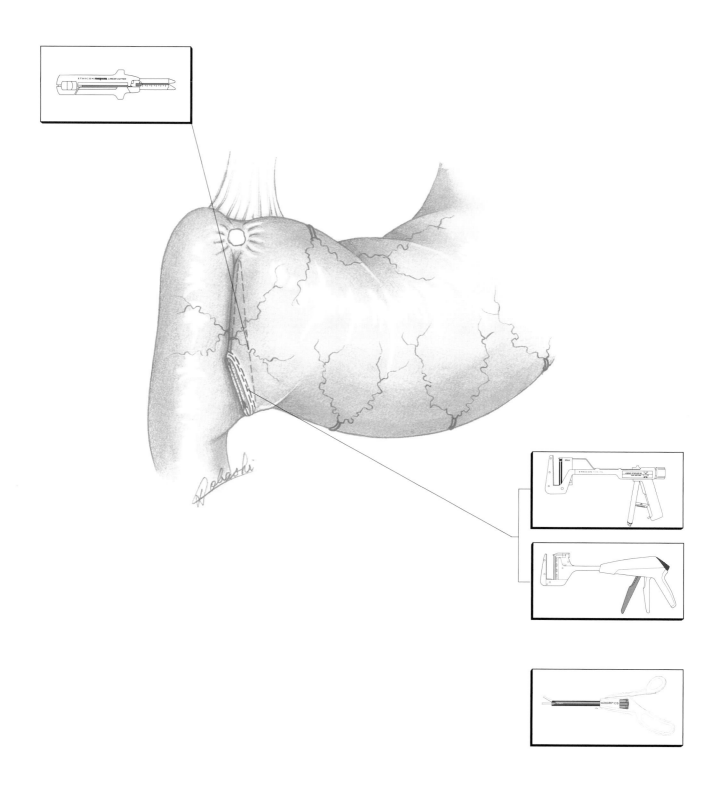

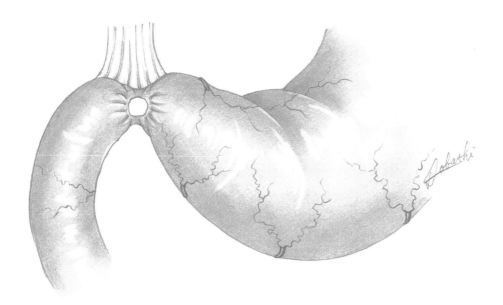

A Kocher maneuver is performed to
mobilize the duodenum.

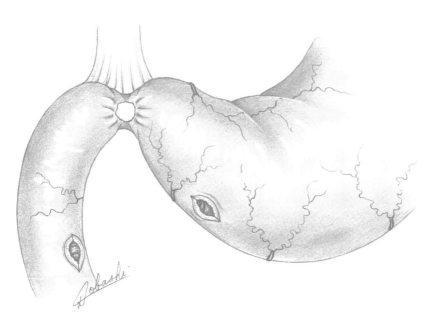

A gastrotomy is made in the region of the greater curvature approximately 5 cm proximal to the pyloric
sphincter. A duodenotomy is made approximately
5 cm distal to the pyloric sphincter. The two openings
are aligned side by side.

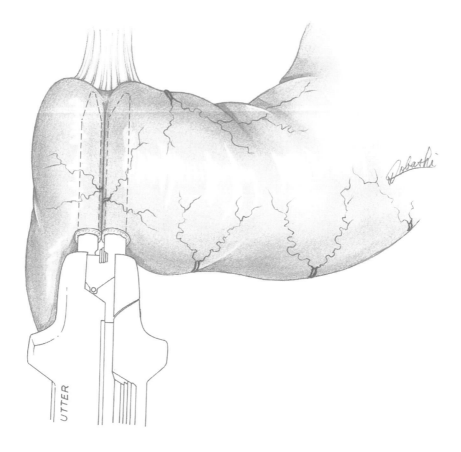

The forks of the linear cutter are inserted into the openings. The instrument is closed and fired, creating the gastroduo-denostomy. The staple line is examined for hemostasis and proper staple formation.

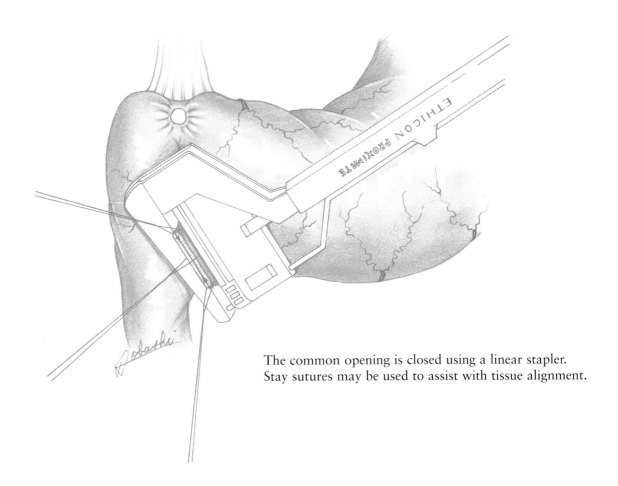

The common opening is closed using a linear stapler.
Stay sutures may be used to assist with tissue alignment.

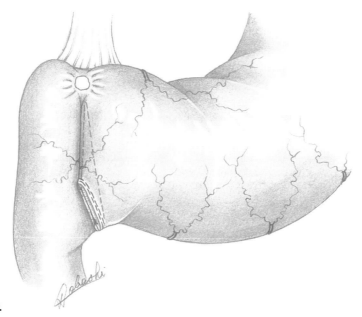

Completed pyloroplasty.

Pyloroplasty

Jaboulay Technique II

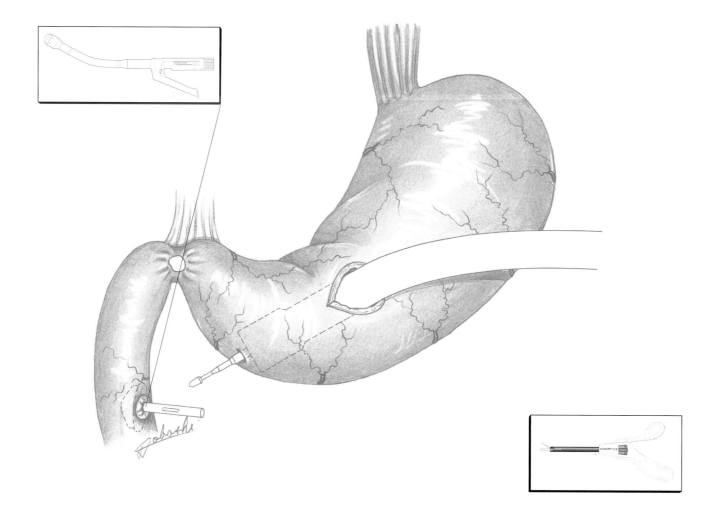

A Kocher maneuver is performed to mobilize the duodenum. A duodenotomy is created 5 cm distal to the pyloric sphincter. (This incision should be large enough to allow the insertion of the anvil of a circular stapler.) A purse-string suture is placed around the duodenotomy, the anvil of the circular stapler inserted, and the purse-string suture tied around the anvil center rod. A gastrotomy is created on the anterior gastric wall. A circular stapler is inserted through the gastrotomy and passed distally. The gastric wall is pierced by the circular stapler's trocar in the region of the greater curvature approximately 5 cm proximal to the pyloric sphincter.

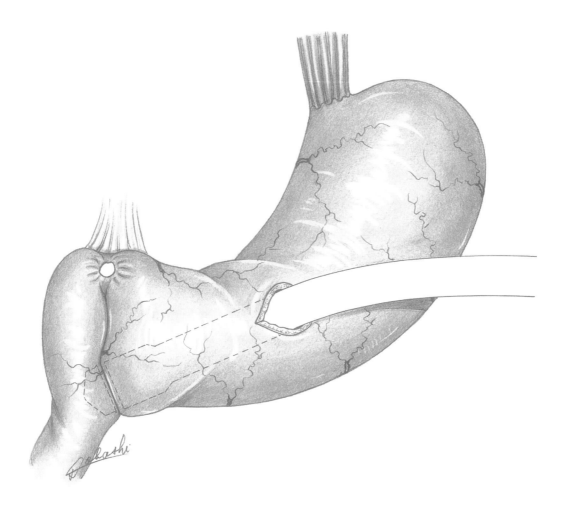

The anvil is attached to the integral trocar, and the circular stapler is closed and fired, creating a side-to-side gastroduodenostomy. After the circular stapler is withdrawn, the tissue donuts are examined for completeness. The donuts should be intact and include all tissue layers. If the donuts are not complete, the anastomosis should be carefully checked for leakage and appropriate repairs made. The gastrotomy is closed using a linear stapler or sutures.

4 Pancreatic Surgery

Pancreaticoduodenectomy and Subtotal Gastrectomy

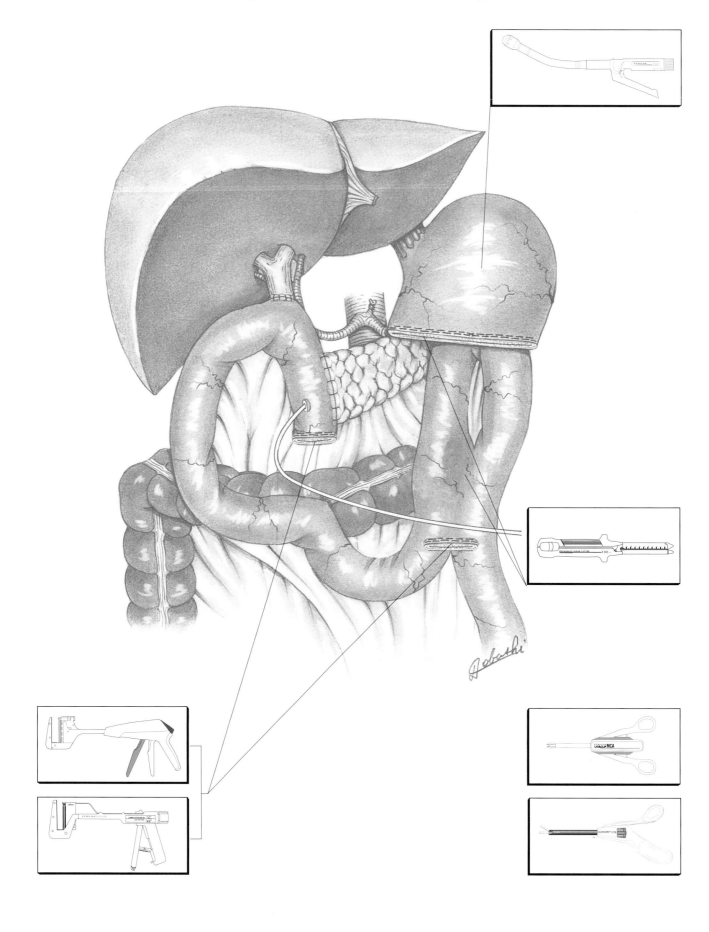

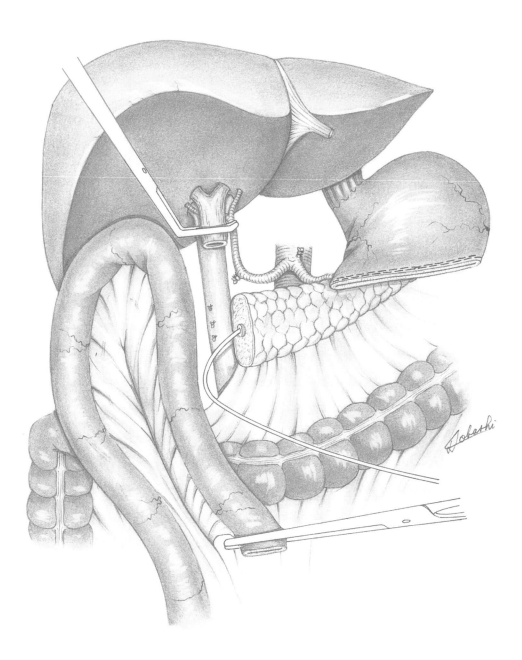

The objective of the procedure is to resect the duodenum and the head of the pancreas. The first step is to mobilize the duodenum and the head of the pancreas with suture ligatures, clips, or the Harmonic Scalpel. A cholecystectomy and a subtotal gastrectomy are performed following the standard techniques. The gastric resection helps visualize the site for the pancreatic transection. The head of the pancreas is transected anterior to the portal vein using a linear stapler. A small catheter or drain may be placed in the major pancreatic duct.

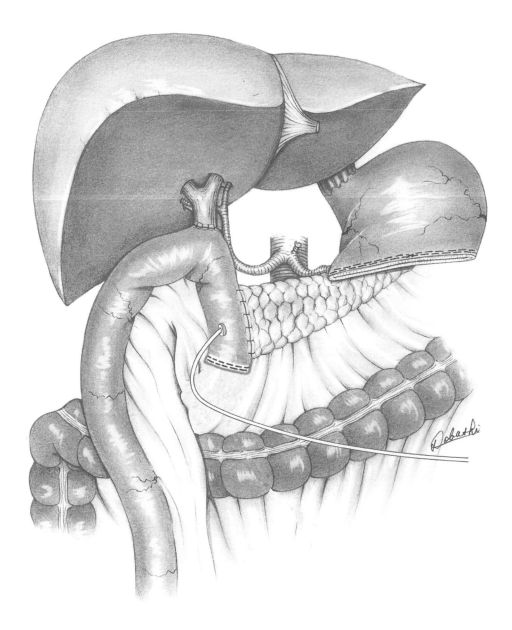

The common bile duct and the pancreatic remnant are anastomosed to the
proximal end of the jejunum with sutures, creating a choledochojejunostomy and
a pancreaticojejunostomy. After the pancreatic catheter is passed through the
jejunal wall, the open proximal end of the jejunum is closed using a linear stapler.

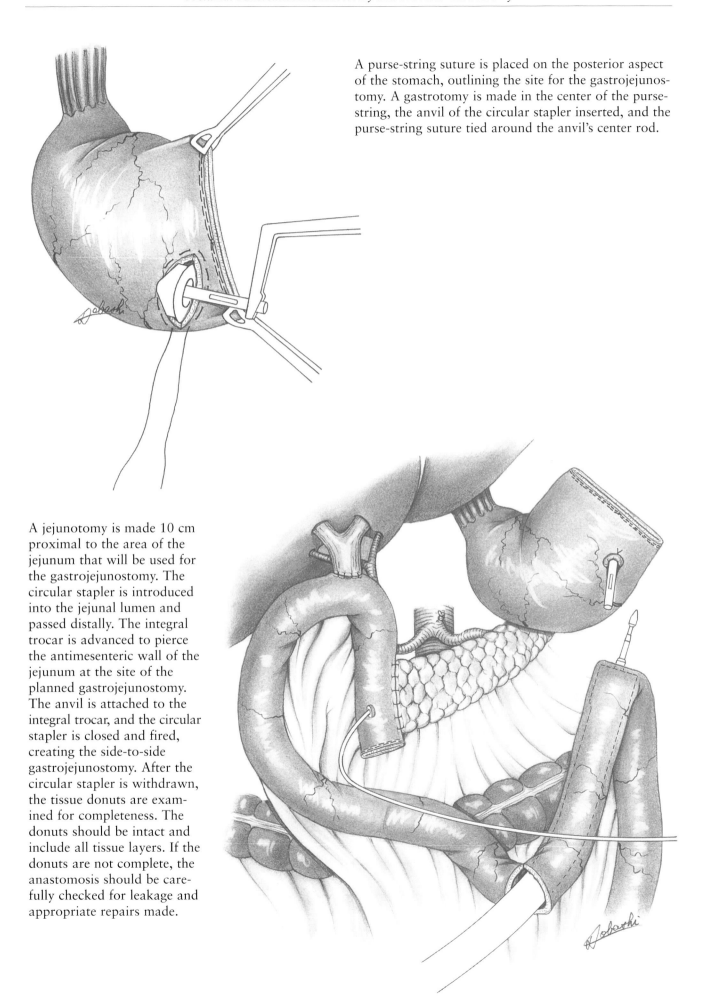

A purse-string suture is placed on the posterior aspect of the stomach, outlining the site for the gastrojejunostomy. A gastrotomy is made in the center of the purse-string, the anvil of the circular stapler inserted, and the purse-string suture tied around the anvil's center rod.

A jejunotomy is made 10 cm proximal to the area of the jejunum that will be used for the gastrojejunostomy. The circular stapler is introduced into the jejunal lumen and passed distally. The integral trocar is advanced to pierce the antimesenteric wall of the jejunum at the site of the planned gastrojejunostomy. The anvil is attached to the integral trocar, and the circular stapler is closed and fired, creating the side-to-side gastrojejunostomy. After the circular stapler is withdrawn, the tissue donuts are examined for completeness. The donuts should be intact and include all tissue layers. If the donuts are not complete, the anastomosis should be carefully checked for leakage and appropriate repairs made.

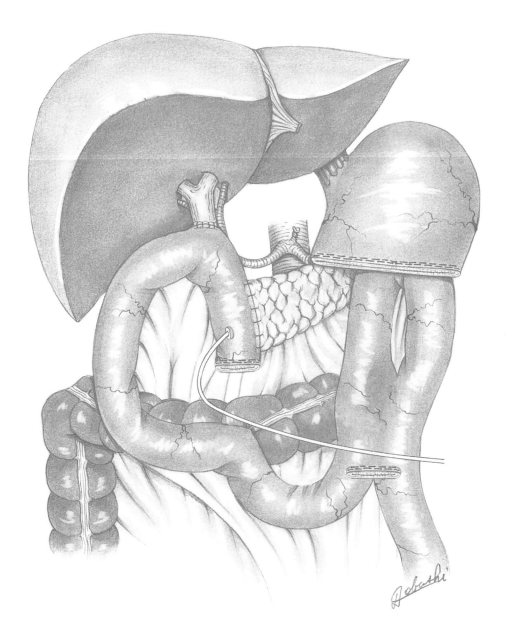

Final result of the procedure after a Braun side-
to-side jejunojejunostomy is created as previously
described.

Distal Pancreatectomy with Splenectomy

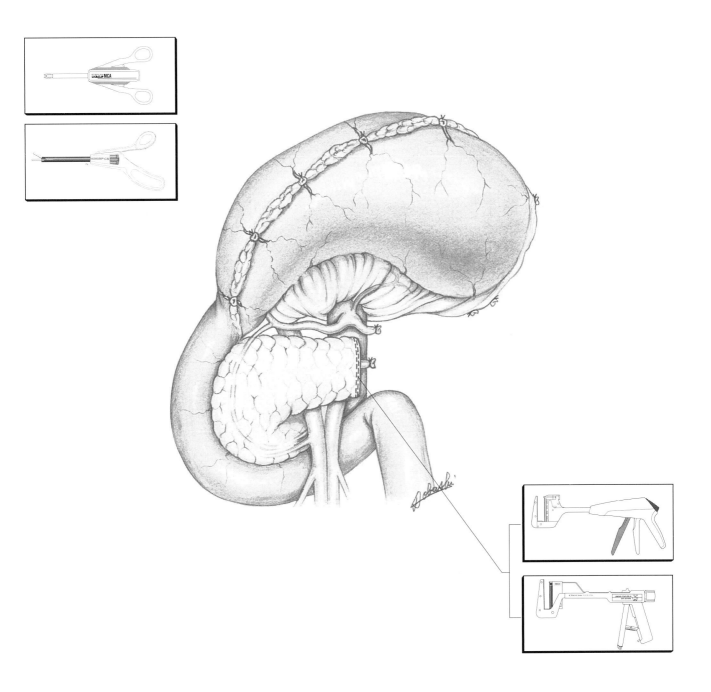

The procedure begins with mobilization of the stomach with suture ligatures, clips, or the Harmonic Scalpel. The spleen is mobilized using suture ligatures, clips, or the Harmonic Scalpel. The splenorenal ligament is exposed, and the splenic artery and vein are ligated and divided. The transection of these vessels is performed in the region where the splenic vein and the superior mesenteric vein merge.

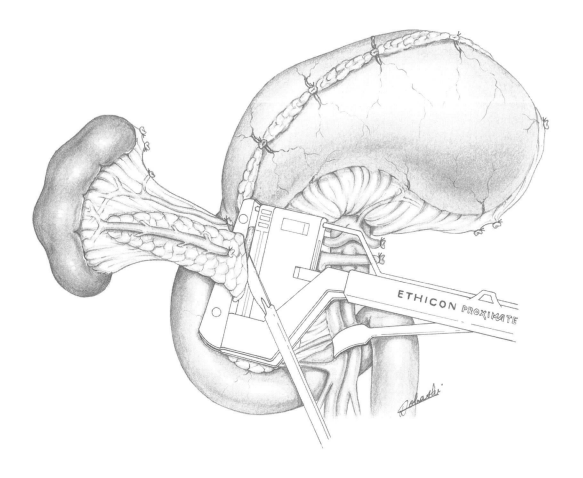

After Mobilization of the Spleen and Distal Pancreas

The distal part of the pancreas is resected with a linear stapler and removed along with the spleen.

Pancreaticocystogastrostomy

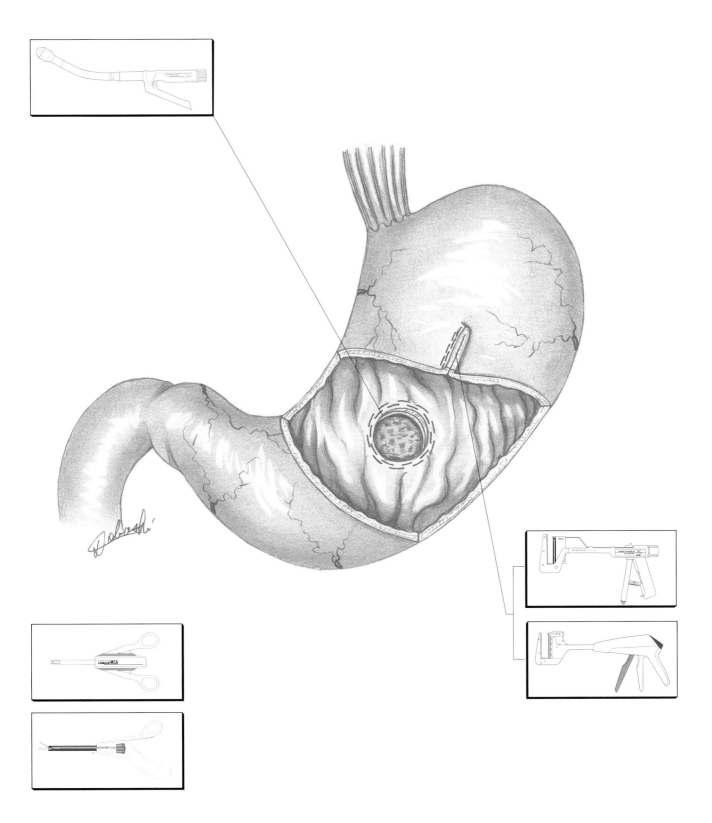

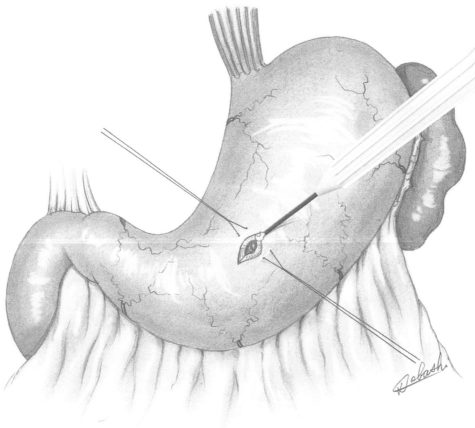

The procedure allows for the creation of an anastomosis between a retrogastric pancreatic cyst and the stomach. An anterior gastrotomy is made with the Harmonic Scalpel. Traction sutures are used to expose the posterior gastric wall.

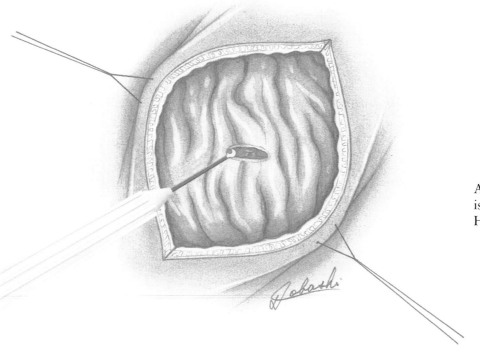

A posterior gastrotomy is performed with the Harmonic Scalpel.

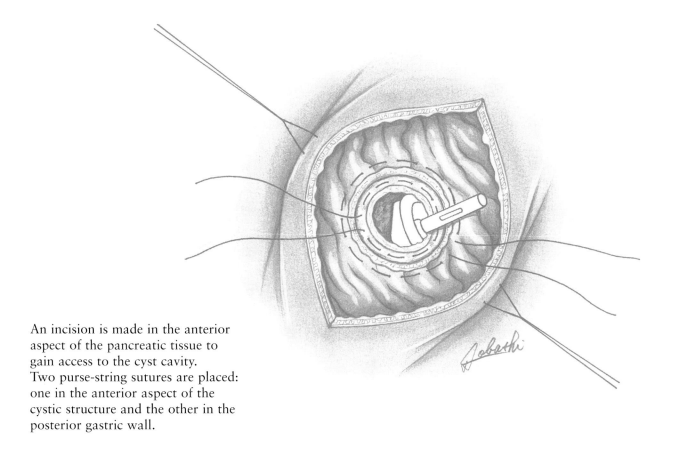

An incision is made in the anterior
aspect of the pancreatic tissue to
gain access to the cyst cavity.
Two purse-string sutures are placed:
one in the anterior aspect of the
cystic structure and the other in the
posterior gastric wall.

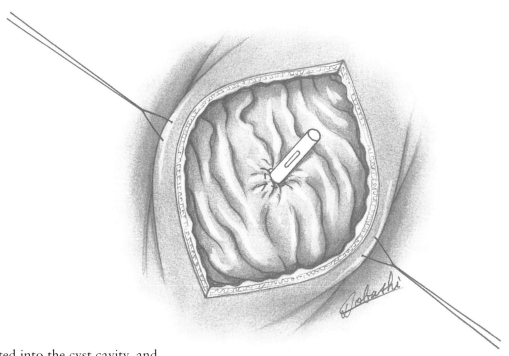

The anvil is inserted into the cyst cavity, and
the two purse-string sutures are tightened
around the tying notch of the anvil center rod.

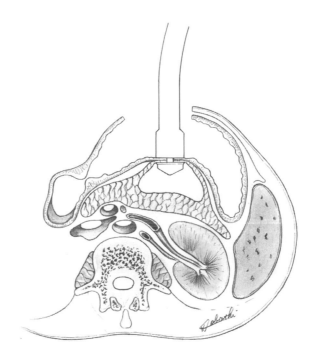

The circular stapler is introduced into the gastric lumen and attached to the previously placed anvil head. The circular stapler is closed and fired, creating the pancreaticocystogastrostomy. After the circular stapler is withdrawn, the tissue donuts are examined for completeness. The donuts should be intact and include all tissue layers. If the donuts are not complete, the anastomosis should be carefully checked for leakage and appropriate repairs made.

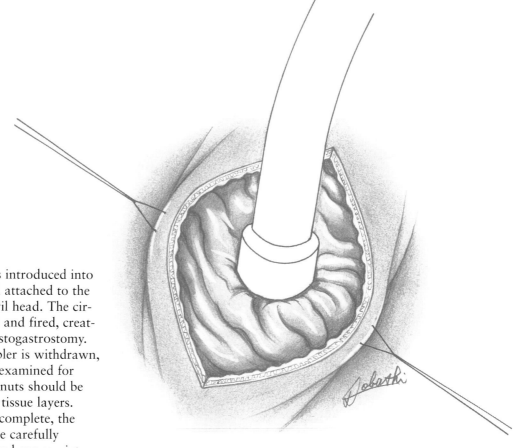

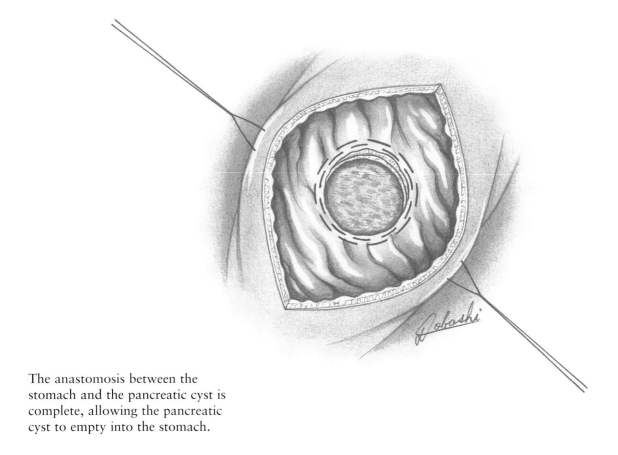

The anastomosis between the stomach and the pancreatic cyst is complete, allowing the pancreatic cyst to empty into the stomach.

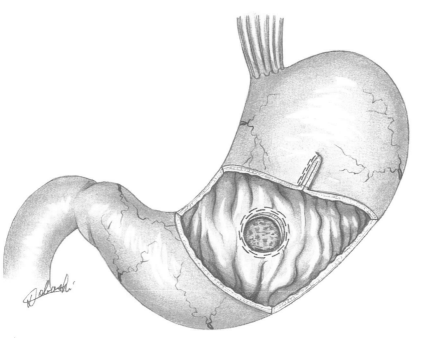

The anterior gastrotomy is closed with a linear stapler.

5 Small Bowel Surgery

Partial Resection of Small Bowel with a Triangulation Anastomosis

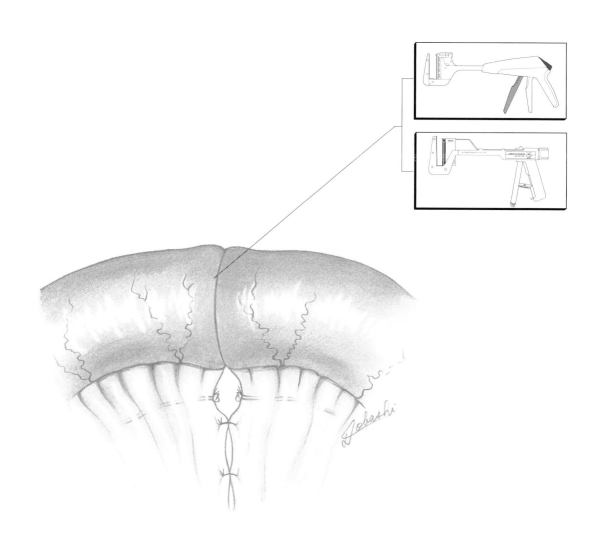

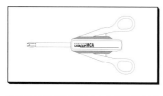

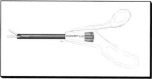

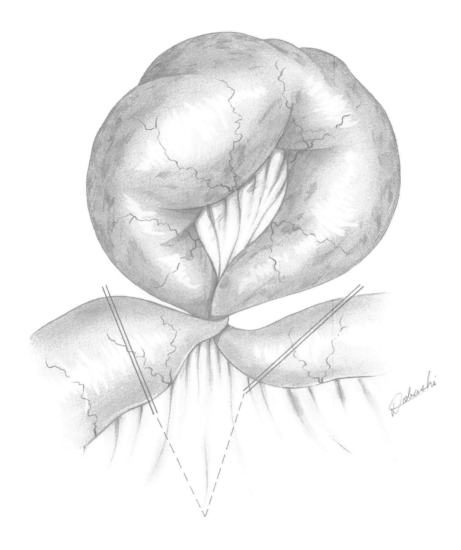

A partial resection of the small bowel may be necessary in
multiple clinical situations. The first step is mobilization of the
involved segments of the small bowel using suture ligatures,
clips, or the Harmonic Scalpel.

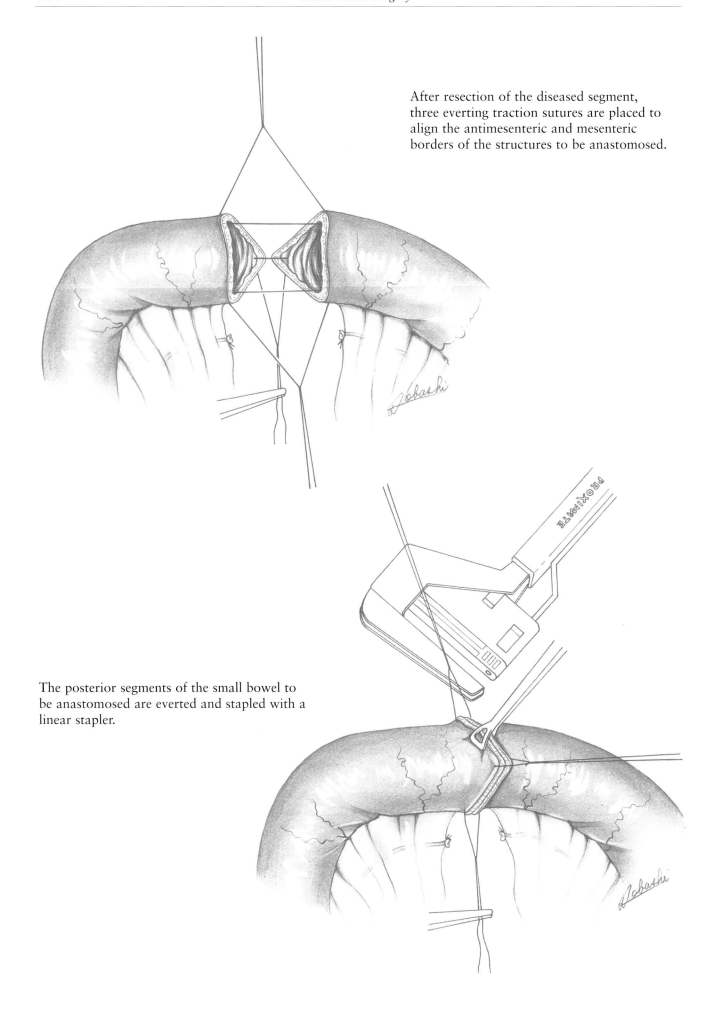

After resection of the diseased segment, three everting traction sutures are placed to align the antimesenteric and mesenteric borders of the structures to be anastomosed.

The posterior segments of the small bowel to be anastomosed are everted and stapled with a linear stapler.

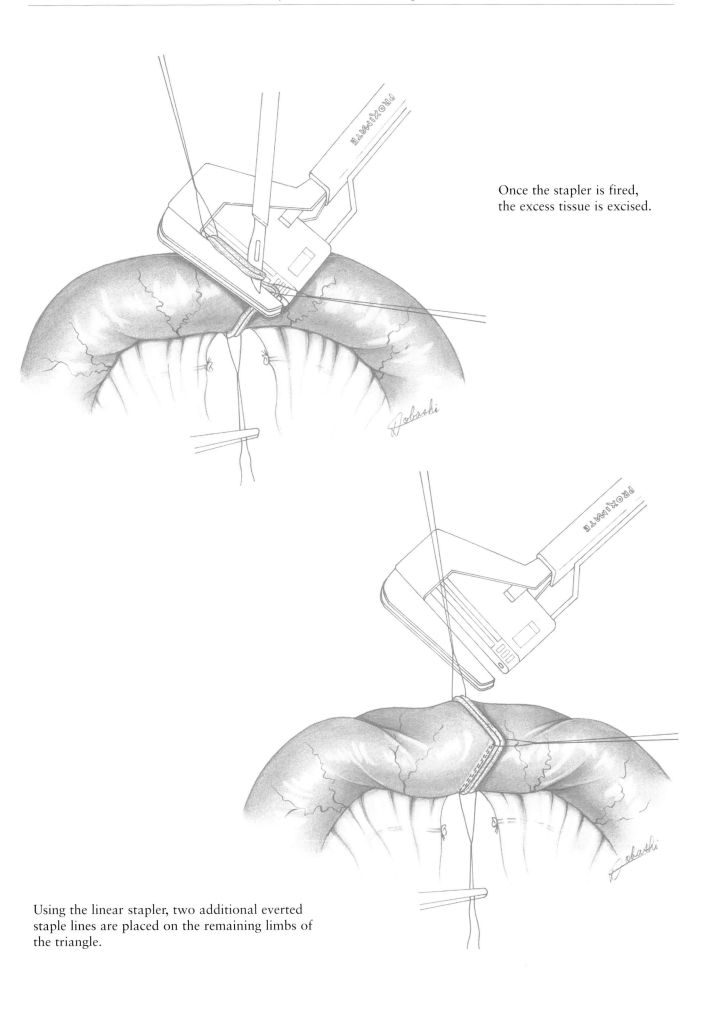

Once the stapler is fired, the excess tissue is excised.

Using the linear stapler, two additional everted staple lines are placed on the remaining limbs of the triangle.

Meckel's Diverticulectomy

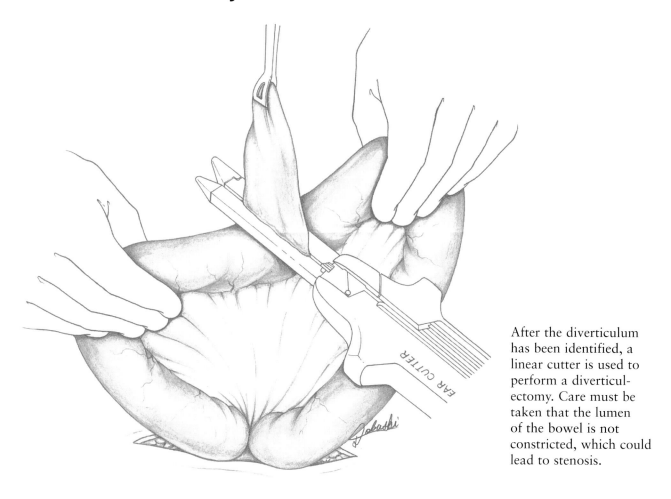

After the diverticulum has been identified, a linear cutter is used to perform a diverticulectomy. Care must be taken that the lumen of the bowel is not constricted, which could lead to stenosis.

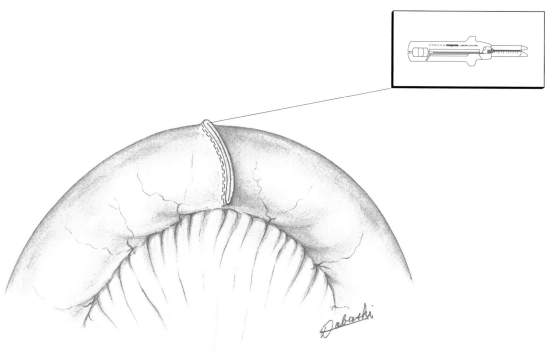

Completed diverticulectomy.

6 Large Bowel Surgery

Appendectomy

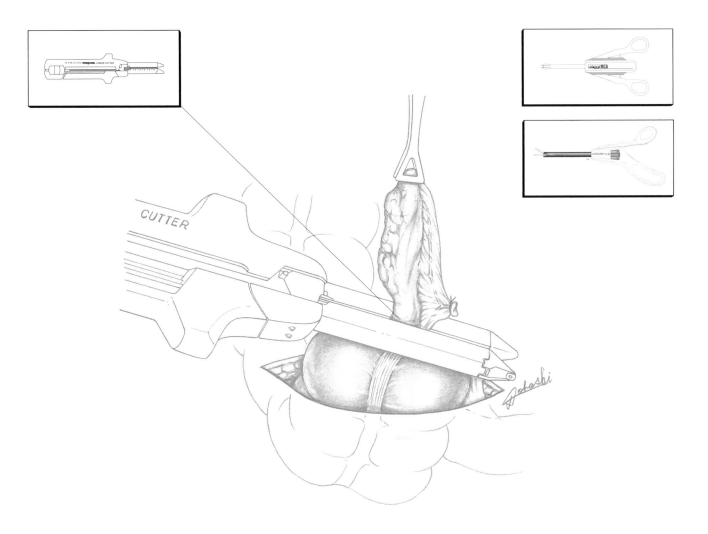

An appendectomy can be performed using the linear stapler or the linear cutter. The procedure involves ligating the mesoappendix with suture ligatures, clips, or the Harmonic Scalpel. Once mobilized, the appendix is transected at its base and removed.

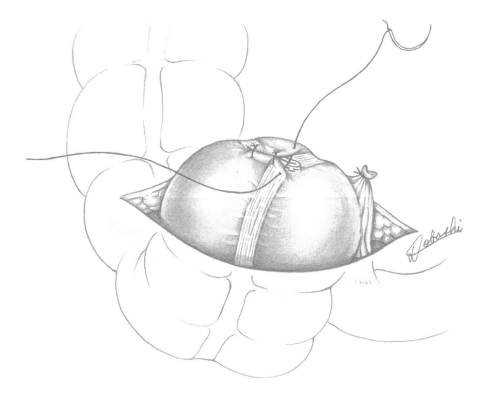

If desired, the stump is inverted with a purse-string suture
or an imbricating interrupted suture.

Bypass of the Right Colon with Side-to-Side Ileocolostomy

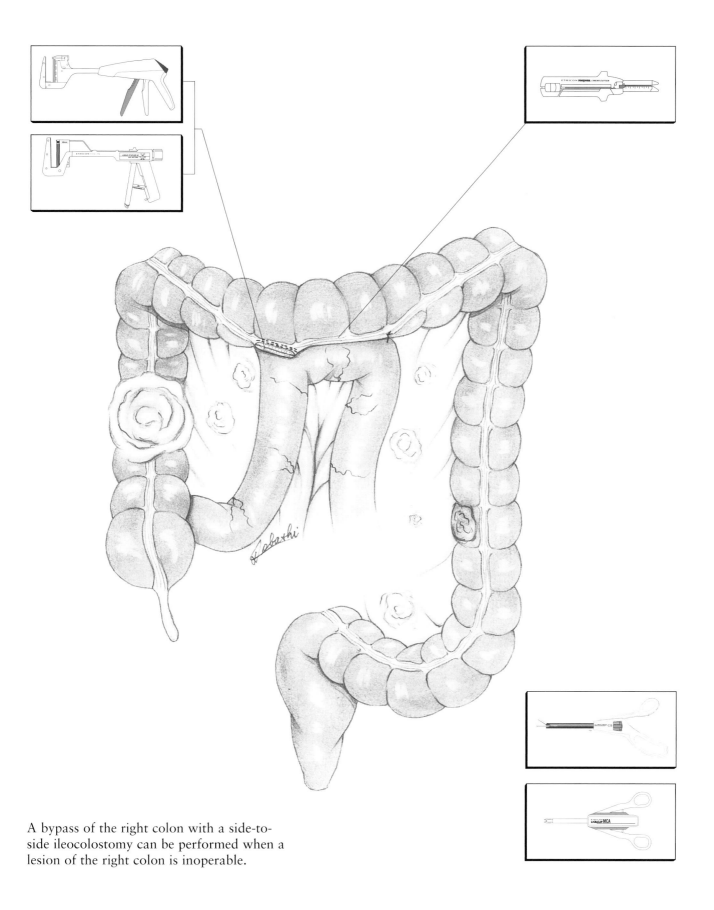

A bypass of the right colon with a side-to-side ileocolostomy can be performed when a lesion of the right colon is inoperable.

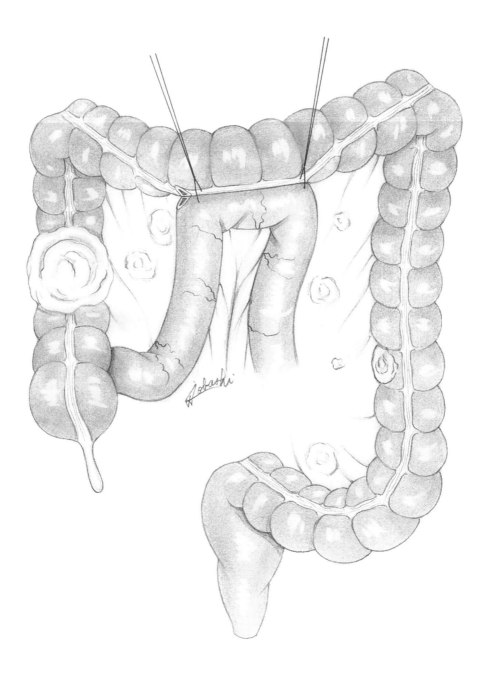

The antimesenteric margins of the transverse colon and
the ileal segment chosen for the bypass are approximated.
Adjacent otomies are created to perform the anastomosis.

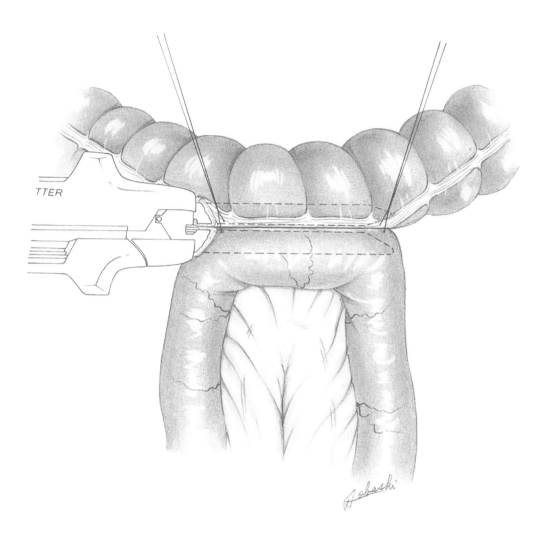

The side-to-side anastomosis is created with a linear cutter.

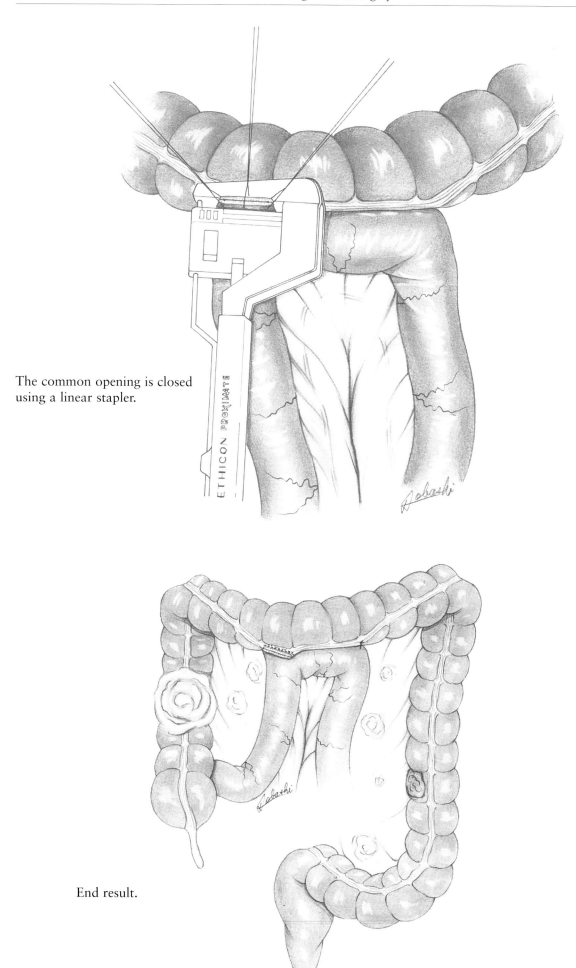

The common opening is closed using a linear stapler.

End result.

Right Hemicolectomy with End-to-Side Ileocolostomy

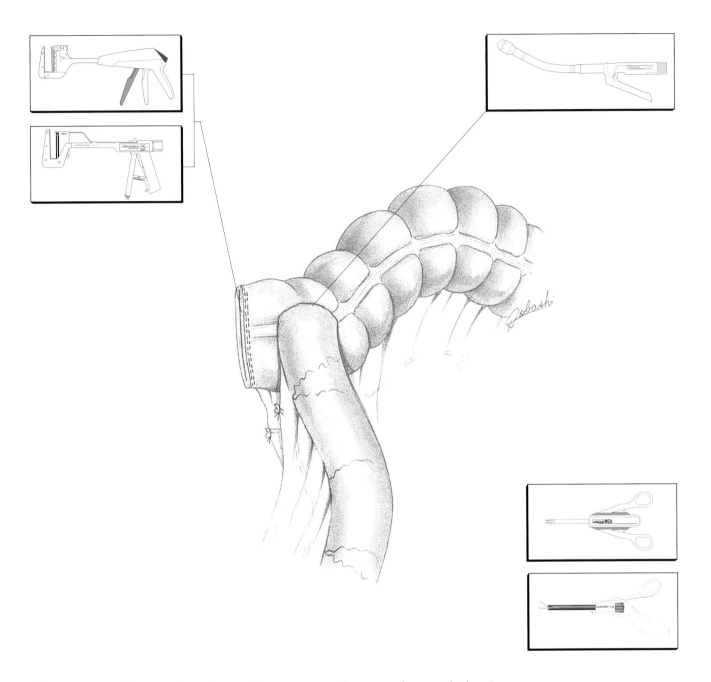

There are several ways of creating an ileotransversecolostomy after a right hemi-colectomy. An end-to-side or a side-to-side anastomosis is the technique most often used. The end-to-side technique is created with a circular stapler.

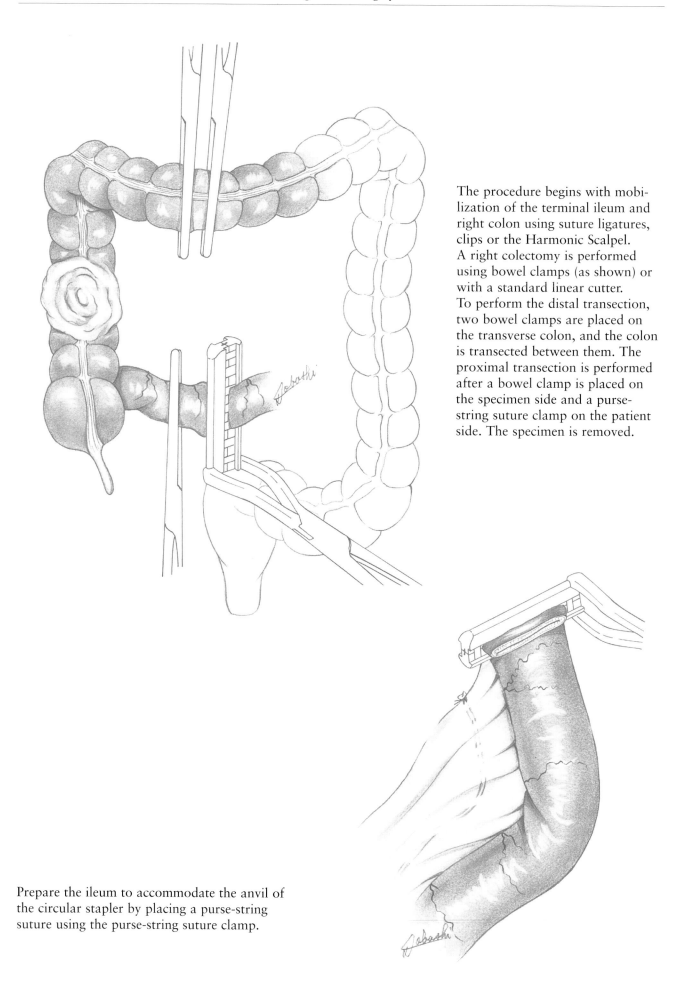

The procedure begins with mobilization of the terminal ileum and right colon using suture ligatures, clips or the Harmonic Scalpel.
A right colectomy is performed using bowel clamps (as shown) or with a standard linear cutter.
To perform the distal transection, two bowel clamps are placed on the transverse colon, and the colon is transected between them. The proximal transection is performed after a bowel clamp is placed on the specimen side and a purse-string suture clamp on the patient side. The specimen is removed.

Prepare the ileum to accommodate the anvil of the circular stapler by placing a purse-string suture using the purse-string suture clamp.

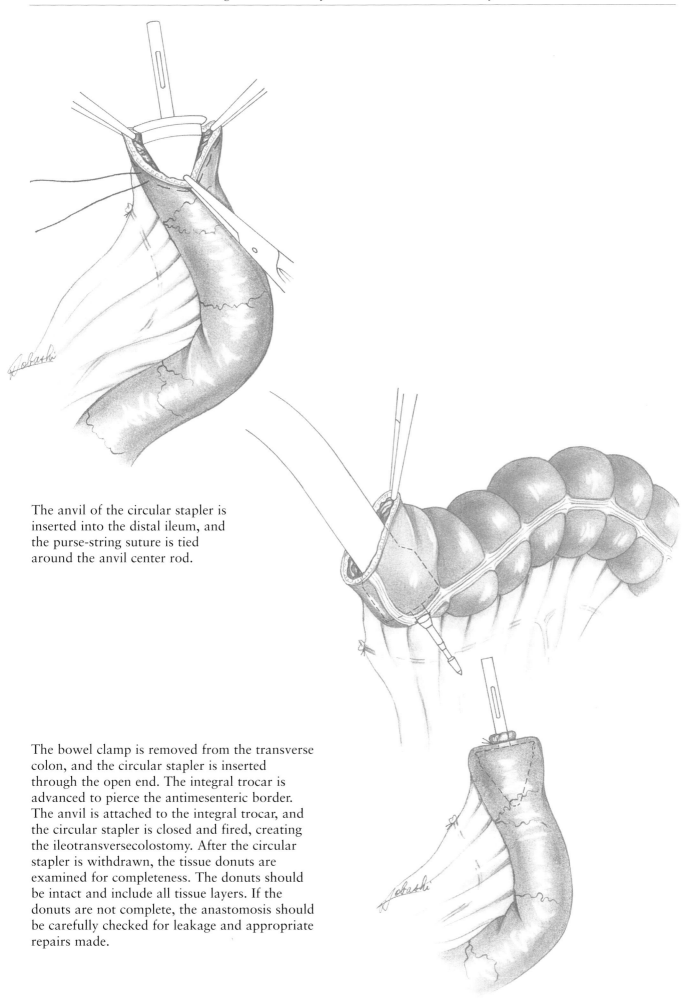

The anvil of the circular stapler is inserted into the distal ileum, and the purse-string suture is tied around the anvil center rod.

The bowel clamp is removed from the transverse colon, and the circular stapler is inserted through the open end. The integral trocar is advanced to pierce the antimesenteric border. The anvil is attached to the integral trocar, and the circular stapler is closed and fired, creating the ileotransversecolostomy. After the circular stapler is withdrawn, the tissue donuts are examined for completeness. The donuts should be intact and include all tissue layers. If the donuts are not complete, the anastomosis should be carefully checked for leakage and appropriate repairs made.

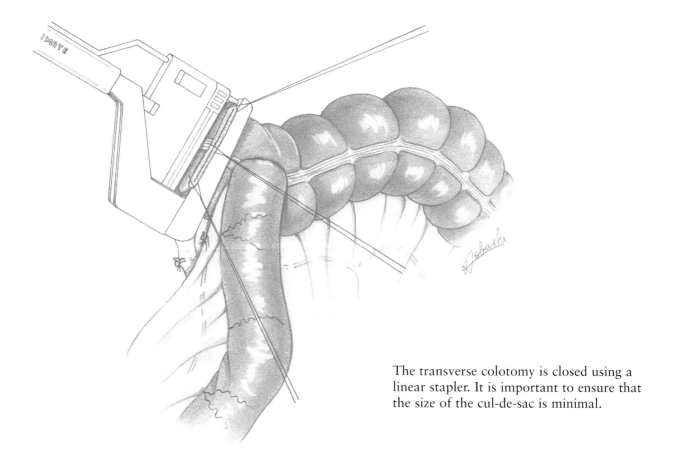

The transverse colotomy is closed using a linear stapler. It is important to ensure that the size of the cul-de-sac is minimal.

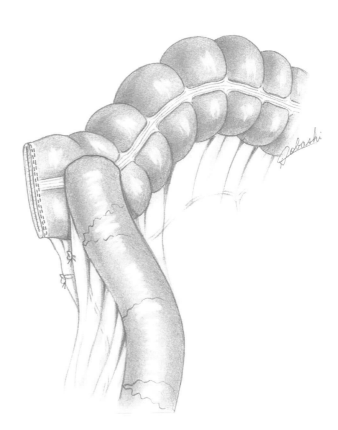

View of the completed anastomosis. The mesenteric defect is closed to avoid potential bowel herniation or torsion.

Right Hemicolectomy with Side-to-Side Ileocolostomy (Functional End-to-End)

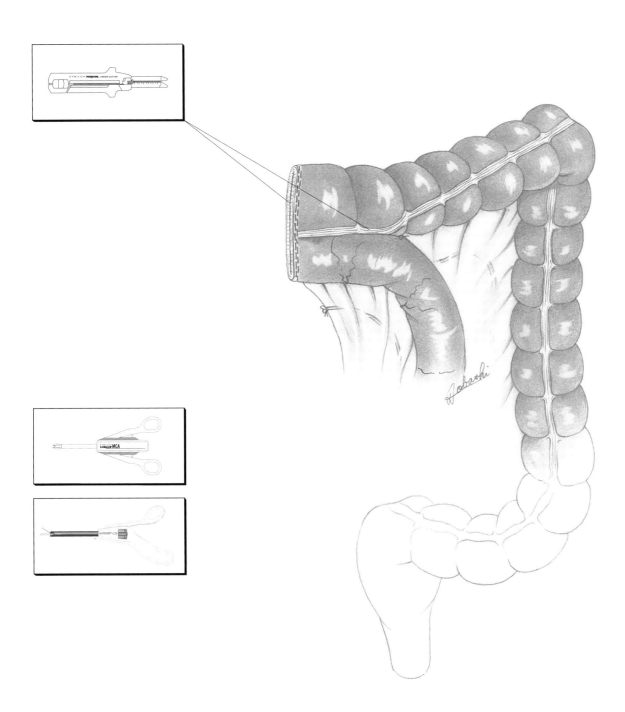

After a right hemicolectomy, bowel continuity is restored by performing a side-to-side ileotransversecolostomy.

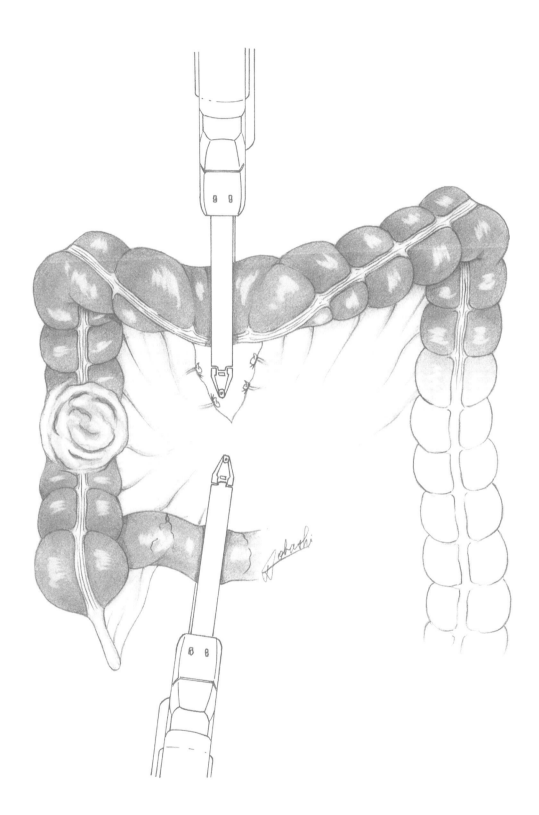

The procedure begins with mobilization of the right
colon using suture ligatures, clips, or the Harmonic
Scalpel. A linear cutter is placed and fired at predefined
points on the ileum and the transverse colon to create
the proximal and distal lines of transection.
The diseased segment is removed.

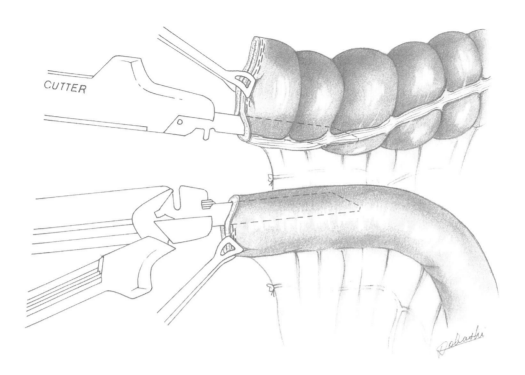

To perform the anastomosis, the antimesenteric borders of the proximal and distal bowel segments are aligned. The corners of the staple lines on the antimesenteric borders are resected with scissors, allowing the forks of the linear cutter to be inserted.

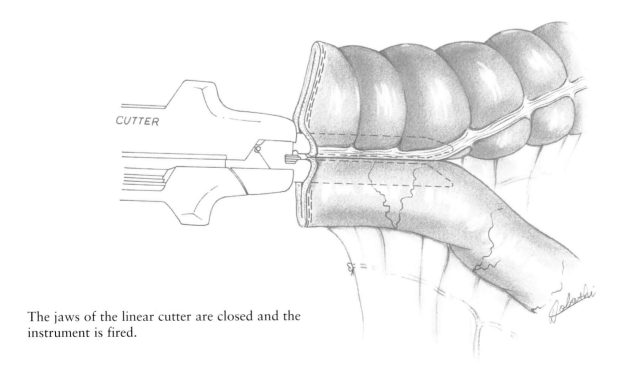

The jaws of the linear cutter are closed and the instrument is fired.

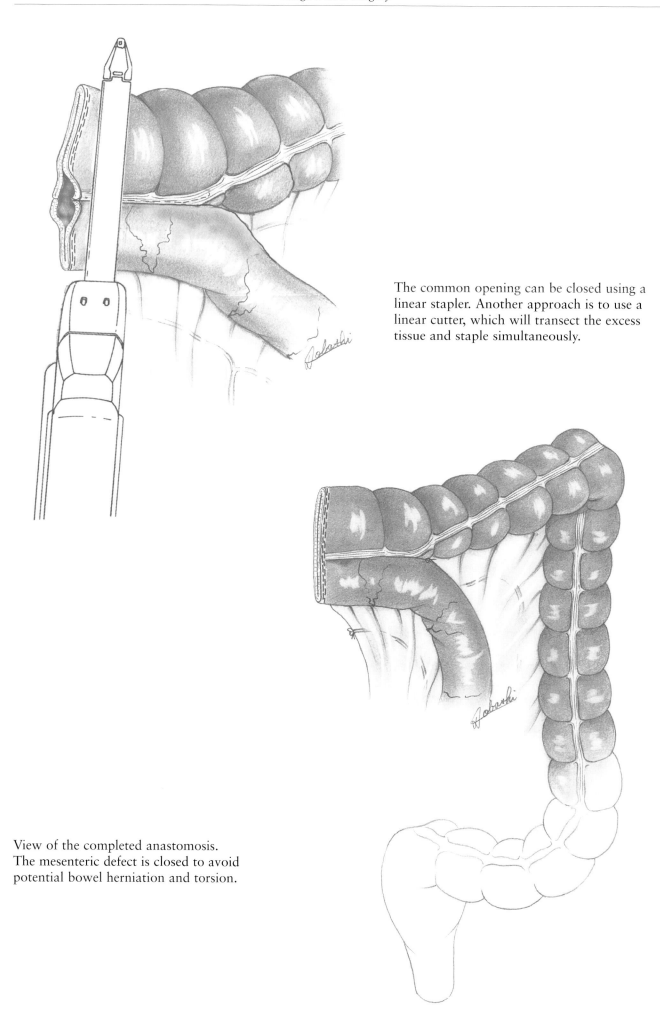

The common opening can be closed using a linear stapler. Another approach is to use a linear cutter, which will transect the excess tissue and staple simultaneously.

View of the completed anastomosis. The mesenteric defect is closed to avoid potential bowel herniation and torsion.

Transverse Colectomy with an End-to-End Anastomosis

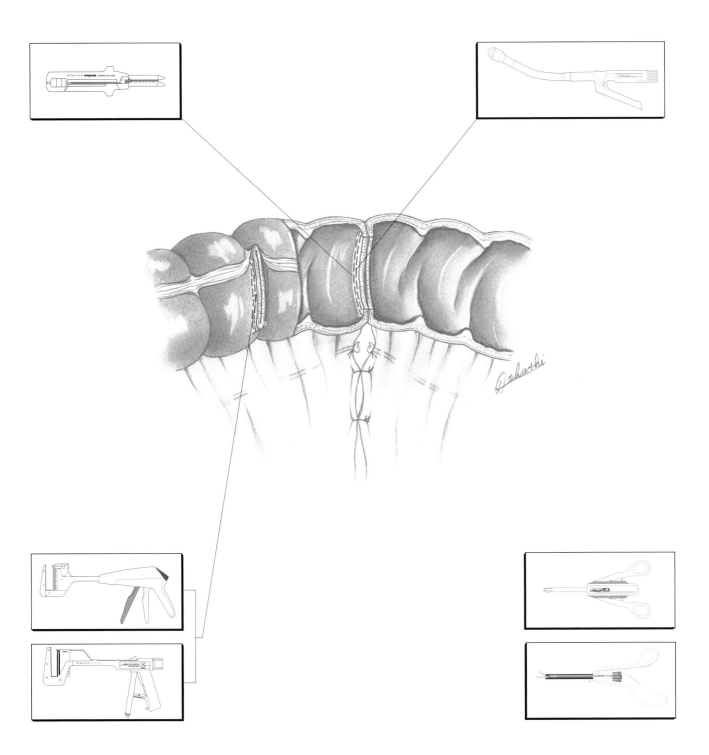

A transverse colectomy is performed. The most frequently used reconstructive methods are an end-to-end or a side-to-side anastomosis. To perform an end-to-end colocolostomy, a colotomy is required to insert the circular stapler.

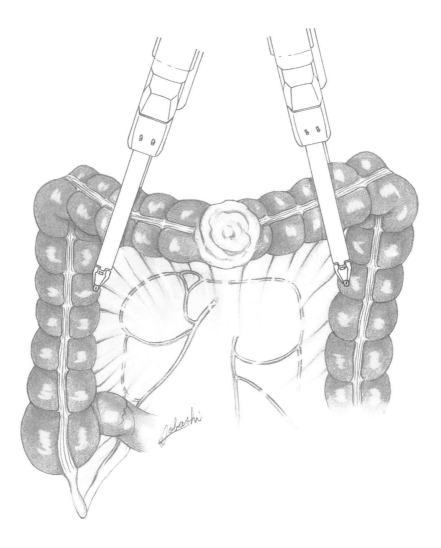

The procedure begins with mobilization of the transverse colon using suture ligatures, clips, or the Harmonic Scalpel. The transverse colectomy is performed with two firings of the linear cutter at the predetermined lines of transection.

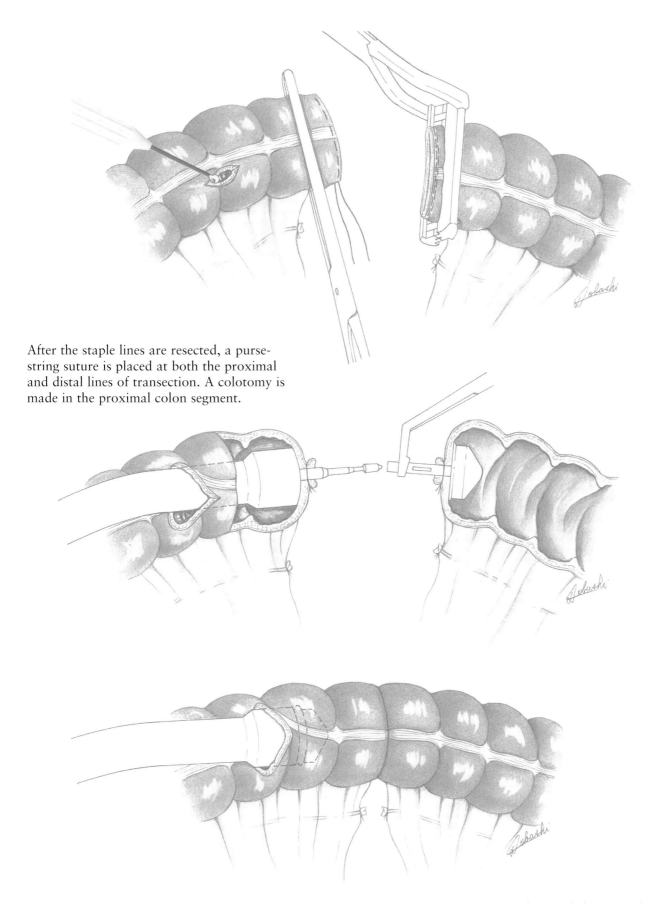

After the staple lines are resected, a purse-string suture is placed at both the proximal and distal lines of transection. A colotomy is made in the proximal colon segment.

The circular stapler is inserted through the colotomy, and the purse-string suture is tied around the integral trocar. The anvil is inserted into the open end of the distal colon segment. The purse-string suture in the distal segment is then tied around the center rod of the anvil. The anvil is attached to the integral trocar, and the circular stapler is closed and fired, creating the colocolostomy.

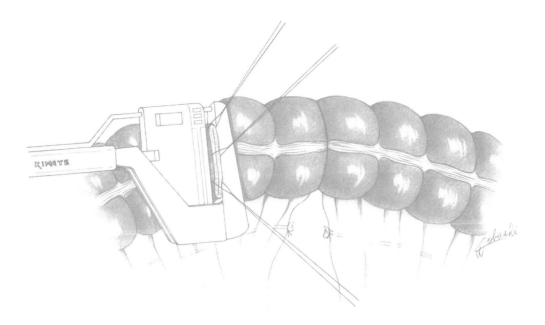

After the circular stapler is withdrawn, the tissue donuts must be examined for completeness. The donuts should be intact and include all tissue layers. If the donuts are not complete, the anastomosis should be carefully checked for leakage and appropriate repairs made. The colotomy is closed using a linear stapler or sutures.

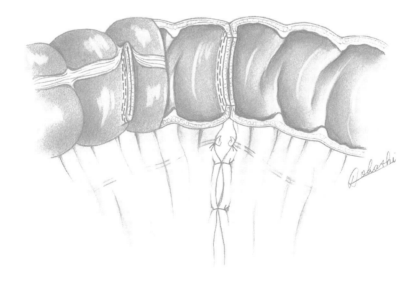

View of the completed anastomosis.
The mesenteric defect is closed.

Transverse Colectomy with Side-to-Side (Functional End-to-End) Anastomosis

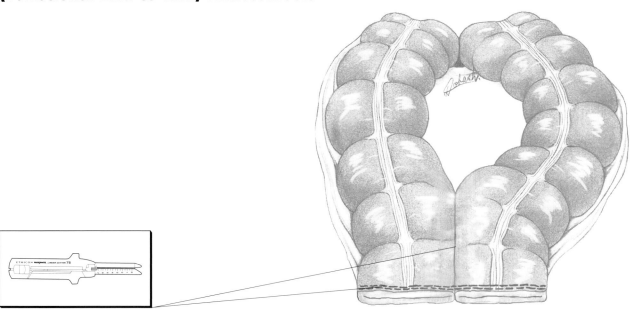

A functional end-to-end anastomosis is created with a linear cutter. The procedure begins with mobilization of the transverse colon with suture ligatures, clips, or the Harmonic Scalpel. A transverse colectomy is performed as previously described.

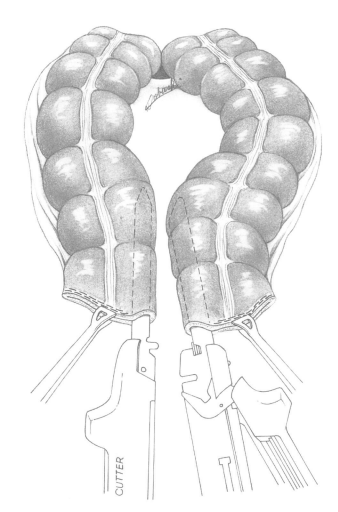

In order to perform the anastomosis, the antimesenteric borders are aligned. The corners of the staple lines on the antimesenteric borders are transected with scissors, which allows the forks of the linear cutter to be inserted.

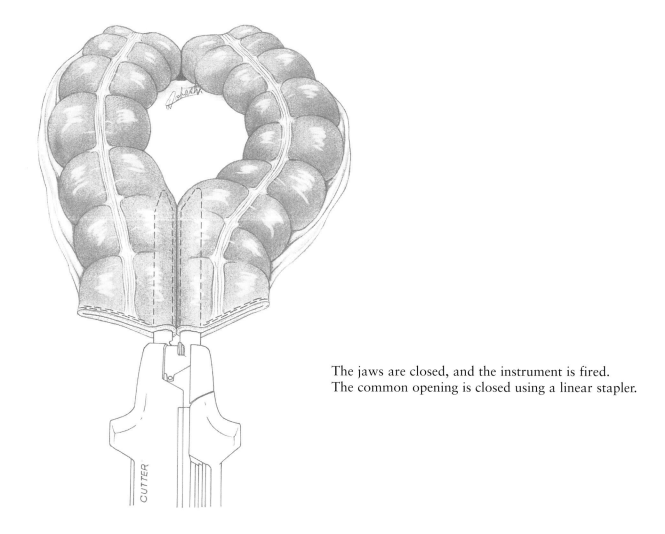

The jaws are closed, and the instrument is fired.
The common opening is closed using a linear stapler.

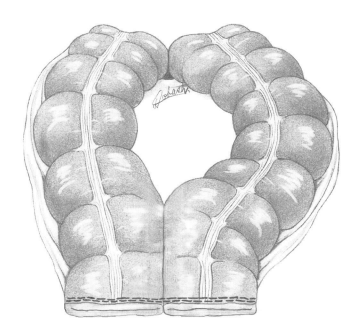

End result of the anastomosis.

Colostomy

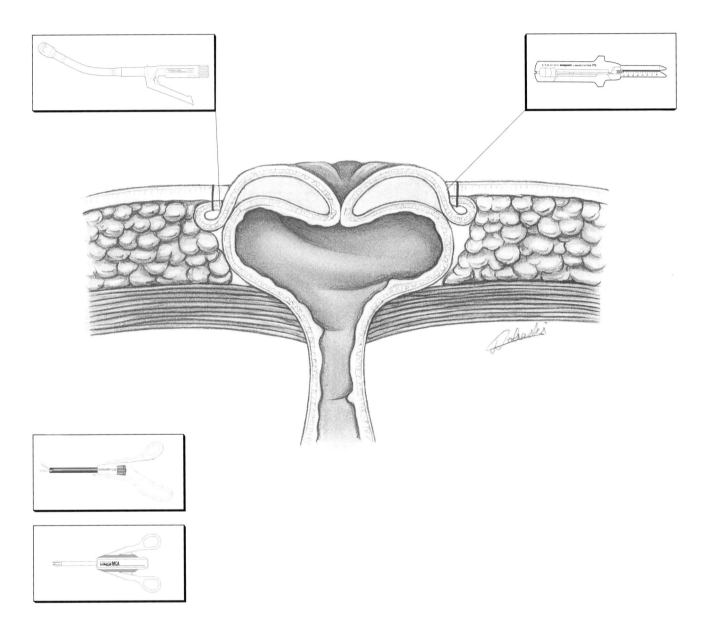

A circular stapler can be used when performing a terminal or end colostomy.
In such cases the distal end of the proximal segment is exteriorized and fixed
to the skin using a wide-diameter stapler to avoid stenosis.

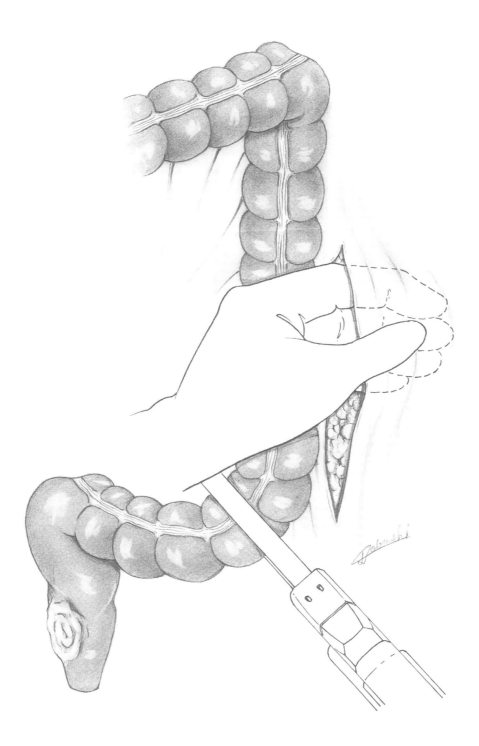

The procedure begins with mobilization of the colon to be
exteriorized, using suture ligatures, clips, or the Harmonic
Scalpel. The colon is transected at a predefined point with
a linear cutter. An opening is made in the abdominal wall
to allow exteriorization of the colon.

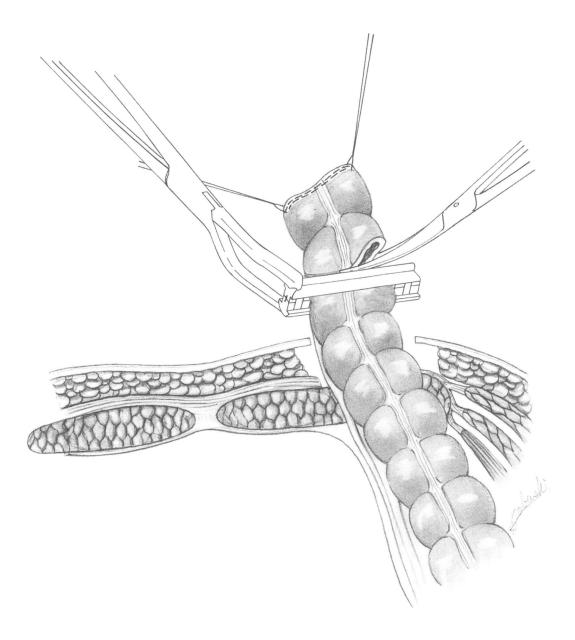

The purse-string suture clamp is placed at a
predefined point on the colon, and a purse-string
suture is placed. The excess tissue is resected
using the cutting edge as a guide.

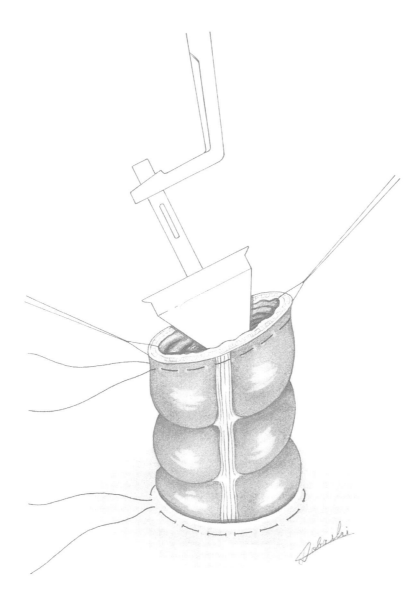

A second purse-string suture is placed at the skin level.
The anvil of the circular stapler is inserted into the colon,
and the purse-string suture is tied around the anvil shaft.

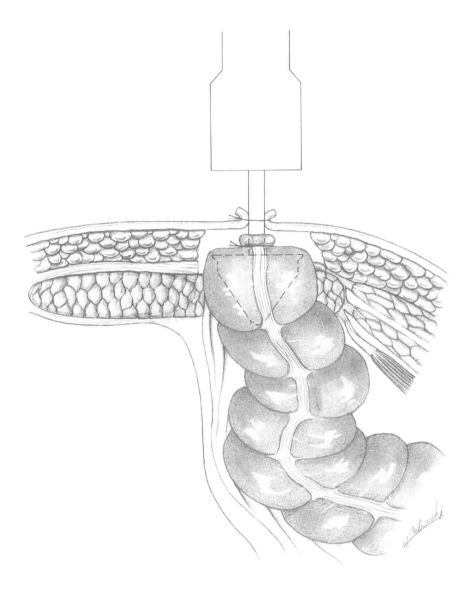

The cutaneous purse-string suture is also tied around the shaft of the anvil. The anvil is attached to the integral trocar, and the circular stapler is closed and fired, creating the colostomy. After the circular stapler is withdrawn, the tissue donuts are examined for completeness. The donuts should be intact and include all tissue layers. If the donuts are not complete, the anastomosis should be carefully checked for leakage and appropriate repairs made.

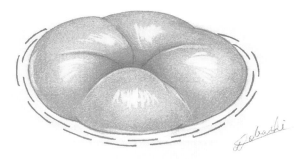

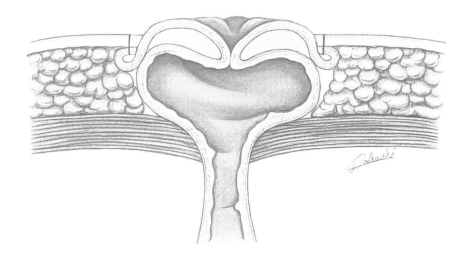

View of the colostomy after the instrument has been fired.

7 Colorectal Surgery

Sigmoidectomy

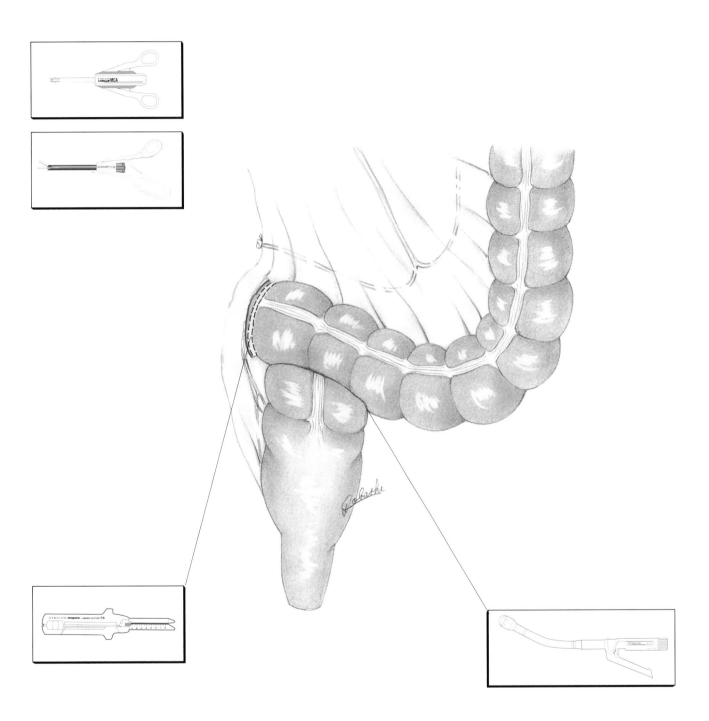

End result after completion of a sigmoidectomy.
The following diagrams illustrate a reconstruction
technique.

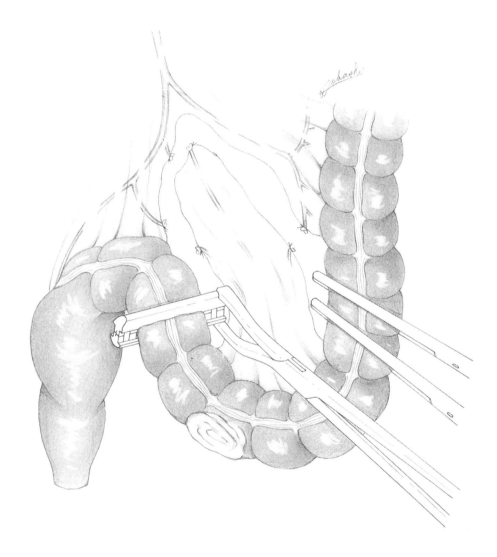

Proximal to the diseased segment, the colon is transected between bowel clamps or with a linear cutter. Distal to the diseased segment, a purse-string suture is placed using a purse-string suture clamp. A bowel clamp is placed on the specimen close to the purse-string suture clamp, and the distal line of transection is created by cutting between them. The specimen containing the diseased segment is then removed.

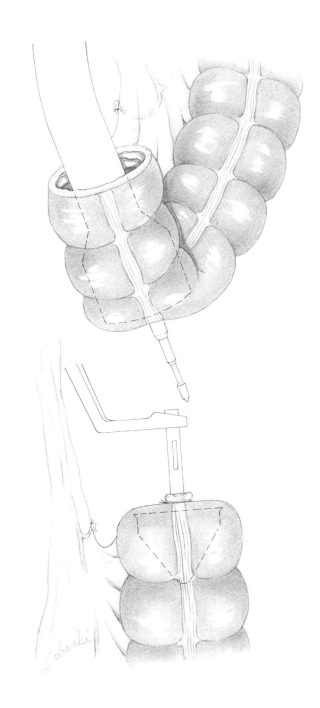

The anvil of an appropriately sized circular stapler is inserted into the
lumen of the proximal end of the distal colonic segment. The purse-string
suture is tied around the anvil center rod.

A circular stapler of an appropriate caliber is inserted into the open distal
end of the proximal colon segment. The integral trocar of the circular
stapler is advanced to pierce the wall of the proximal segment. The anvil is
attached to the integral trocar, and the circular stapler is closed and fired,
creating the side-to-end colocolostomy.

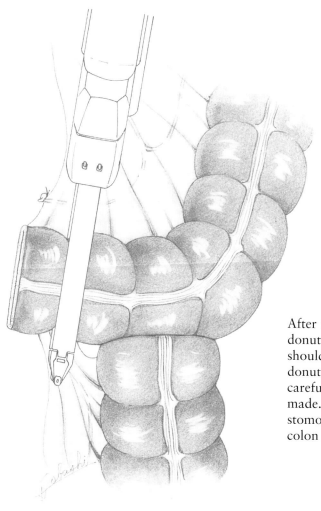

After the circular stapler is withdrawn, the tissue donuts are examined for completeness. The donuts should be intact and include all tissue layers. If the donuts are not complete, the anastomosis should be carefully checked for leakage and appropriate repairs made. A linear cutter is applied 2–3 cm from the anastomosis, so that the redundant portion of proximal colon is excised.

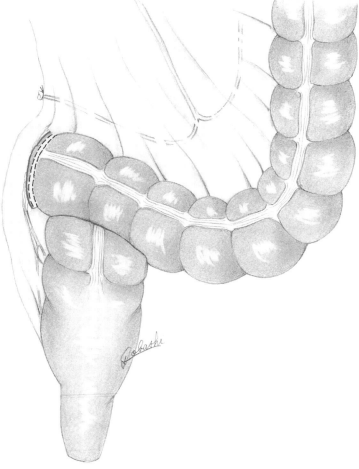

Low Anterior Resection

End-to-End Anastomosis

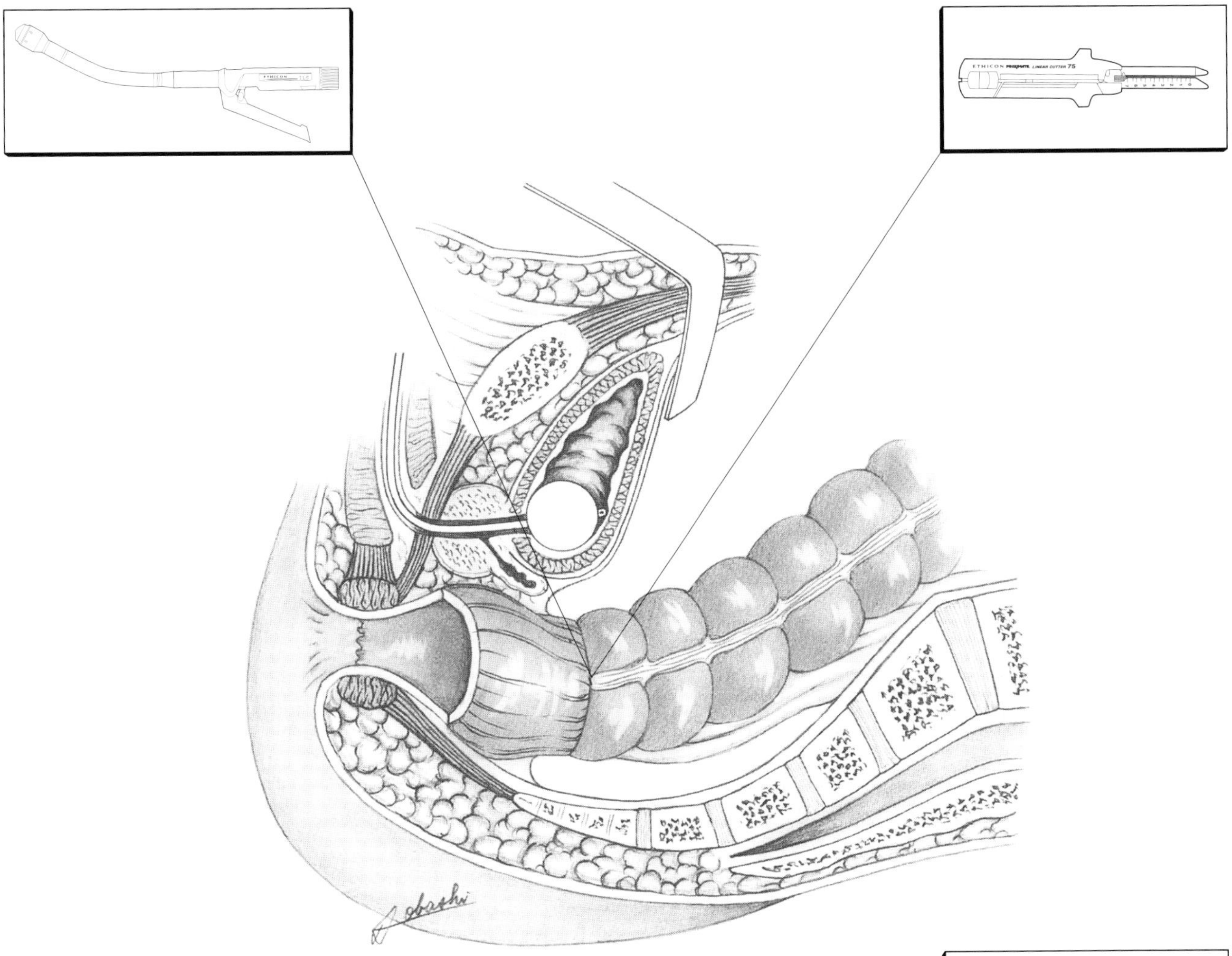

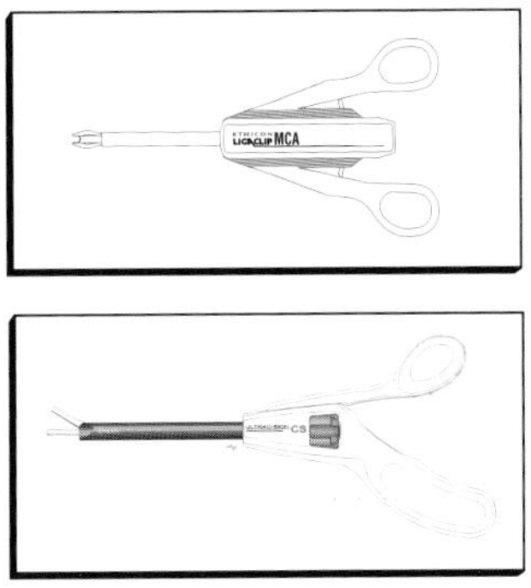

The diagrams illustrate the end-to-end reconstruction technique following a low anterior resection.

The procedure begins with mobilization of the colon to be resected using suture ligatures, clips, or the Harmonic Scalpel. The proximal line of transection is created with a linear cutter. A purse-string suture clamp is placed distal to the diseased segment. Another purse-string suture clamp is placed on the proximal colon proximal and adjacent to the staple line.

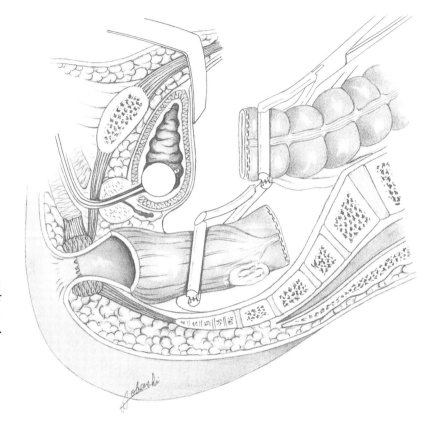

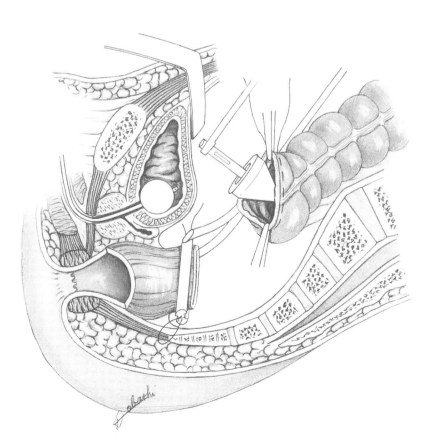

Purse-string sutures are placed in both the proximal and distal segments. Cutting between a bowel clamp and the distal purse-string suture clamp creates the distal line of transection. The diseased segment is then removed. Excess tissue is resected along the cutting guide of the purse-string suture clamps. In the proximal segment, this excess tissue will also include the proximal staple line. After the proximal colon is dilated with sizers, the anvil is inserted into its lumen, and the purse-string suture is tied around the anvil center rod.

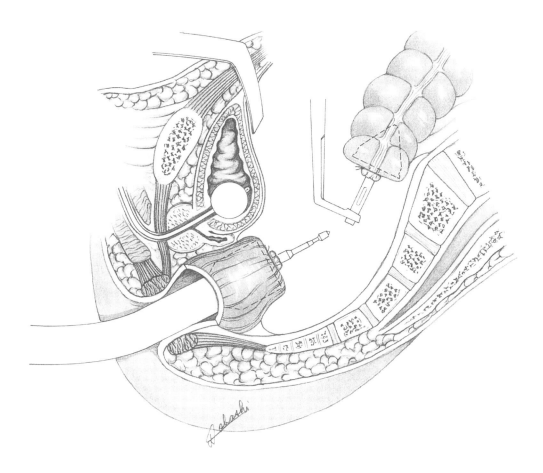

The circular stapler is inserted transanally. After the trocar has been extended, the distal purse-string suture is tied around its base. The anvil is attached to the integral trocar and the circular stapler is closed and fired, creating a colo-proctostomy. After the circular stapler is withdrawn, the tissue donuts are examined for completeness. The donuts should be intact and include all tissue layers. If the donuts are not complete, the anastomosis should be carefully checked for leakage and appropriate repairs made.

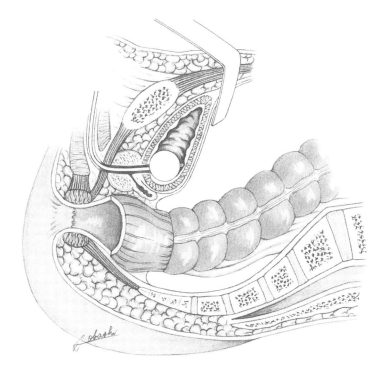

Low Anterior Resection

Double Stapling Technique

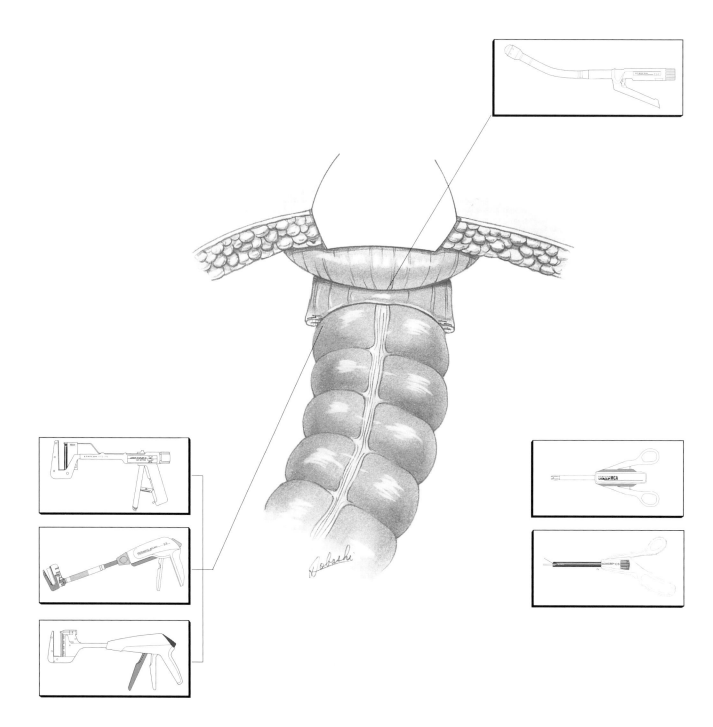

The diagram above illustrates the Knight-Griffen technique, used in cases where construction of the distal purse-string presents difficulties, and when the dimensions of the proximal colon and rectal stump differ.

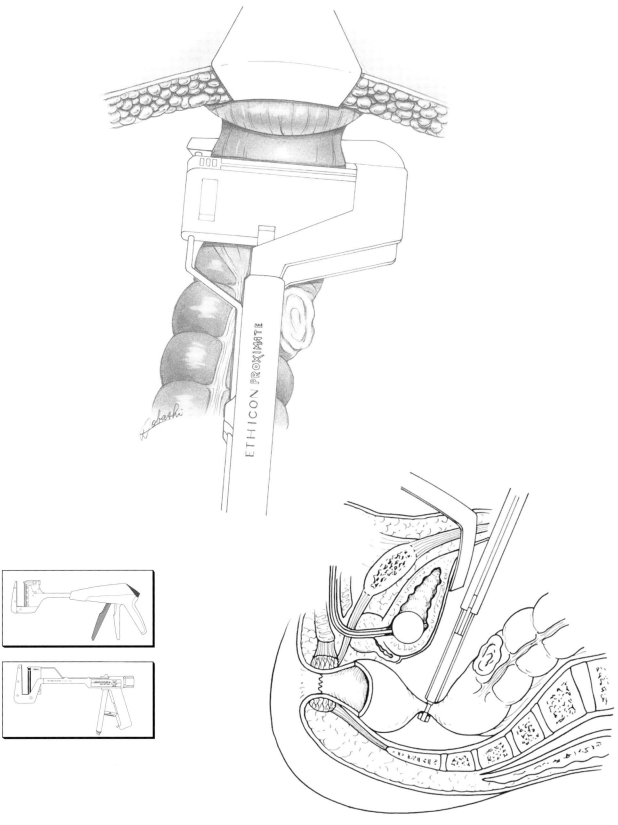

The diseased segment is mobilized using suture ligatures, clips, or the
Harmonic Scalpel. A linear cutter or a Compact Flex is placed below
the diseased segment.

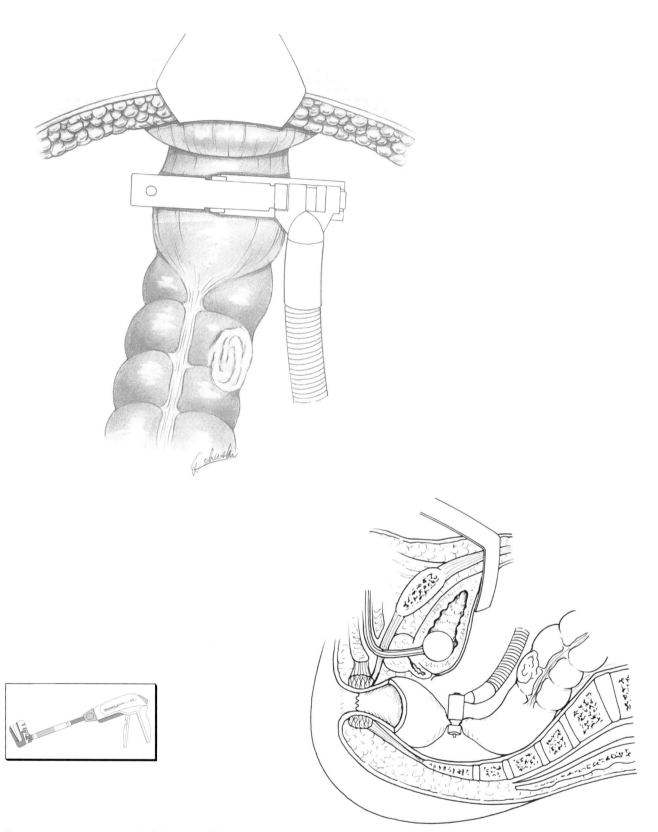

In some patients a stapled closure of the rectal stump is
facilitated by the use of an articulating linear stapler with
a flexible shaft.

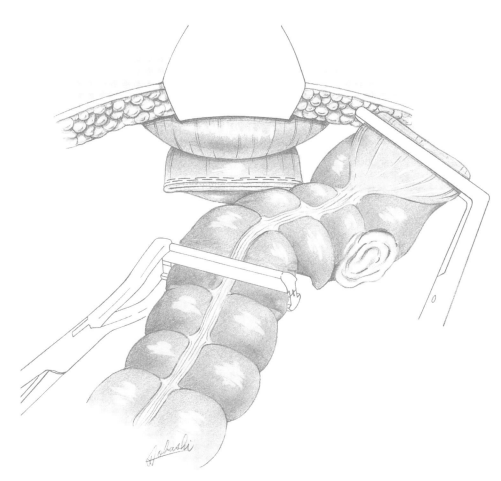

The distal staple line is created with either the articulating linear cutter or the articulating linear stapler.

If an articulating linear stapler is used, a right angle clamp is placed across the bowel proximal to the stapler. The bowel is then transected along the cutting guide of the linear stapler. A purse-string suture clamp is placed proximal to the diseased segment.

The bowel is then transected along the cutting guide of the purse-string suture clamp. The specimen containing the diseased segment is then removed.

Using the purse-string suture clamp, a purse-string suture is placed at the distal end of the proximal colonic segment. The anvil of the circular stapler is inserted into the proximal colonic segment, and the purse-string is closed tightly around its rod. The circular stapler is inserted transanally into the rectal stump.

The integral trocar is advanced so that it pierces the anterior wall of the rectal stump as close to the staple line as possible.

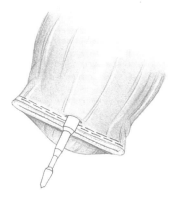

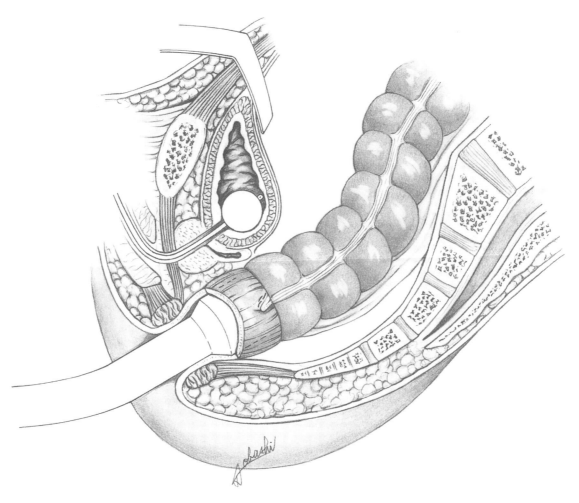

The anvil is attached to the integral trocar, and the circular stapler is closed and fired, creating the coloproctostomy. After the circular stapler is withdrawn, the tissue donuts are examined for completeness. The donuts should be intact and include all tissue layers. If the donuts are not complete, the anastomosis should be carefully checked for leakage and appropriate repairs made.

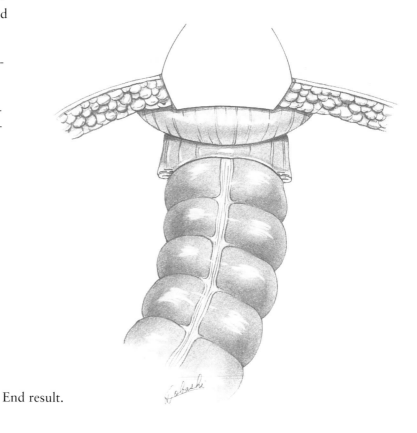

End result.

Low Anterior Resection

Duhamel Procedure

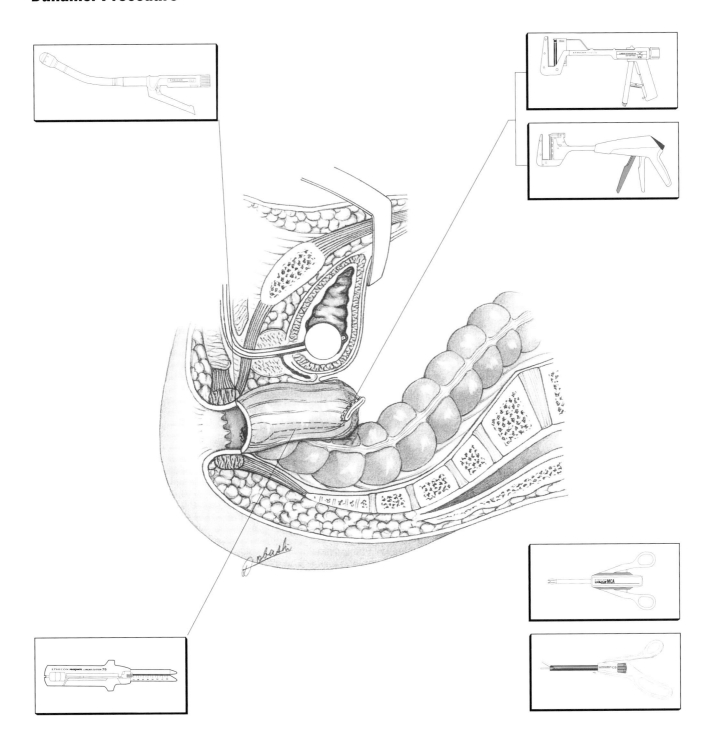

The diagram illustrates the Duhamel procedure, which is indicated for children suffering from Hirschsprung's disease (congenital toxic megacolon).

The diseased segment of the colon is mobilized with suture ligatures, clips, or the Harmonic Scalpel. A linear stapler is applied distal to the diseased segment to create the distal line of transection. The proximal line of transection is created with a linear cutter. The diseased segment is removed.

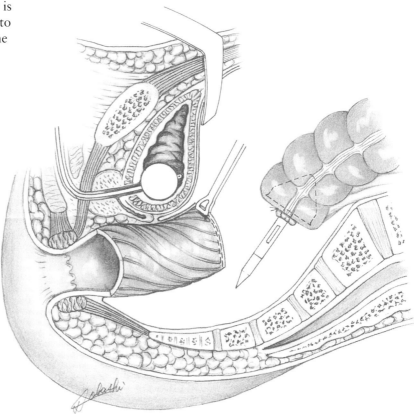

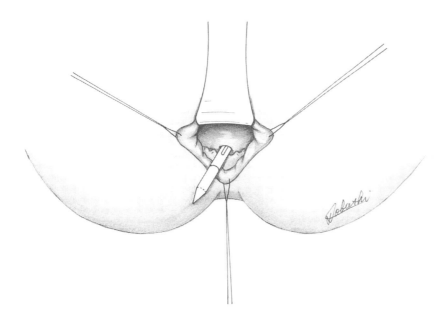

After excising the staple line, a purse-string suture is placed at the distal end of the proximal colon. The anvil of the circular stapler is introduced into the lumen of the distal end of the proximal segment, and the purse-string suture is tied around the anvil rod. The sharp anvil accessory tip is attached to the anvil. The tip of the anvil rod assembly is directed to pierce the posterior wall of the rectum 1–1.5 cm superior to the dentate line.

The sharp anvil rod accessory is detached from the anvil rod. The anvil is attached to the integral trocar tip, and the circular stapler is closed and fired, creating the end-to-side coloproctostomy. After the circular stapler is withdrawn, the tissue donuts are examined for completeness. The donuts should be intact and include all tissue layers. If the donuts are not complete, the anastomosis should be carefully checked for leakage and appropriate repairs made.

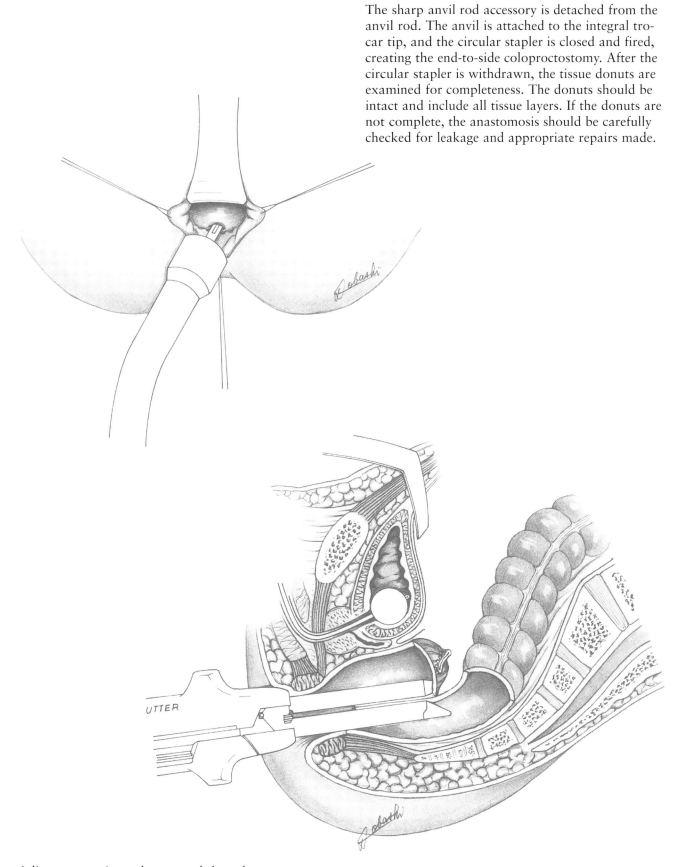

A linear cutter is used to extend the coloproctostomy in order to create a reservoir.

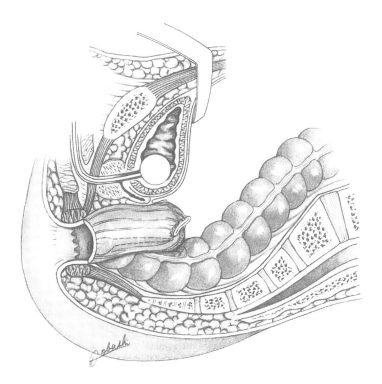

End result.

Colectomy: J-Pouch (1)

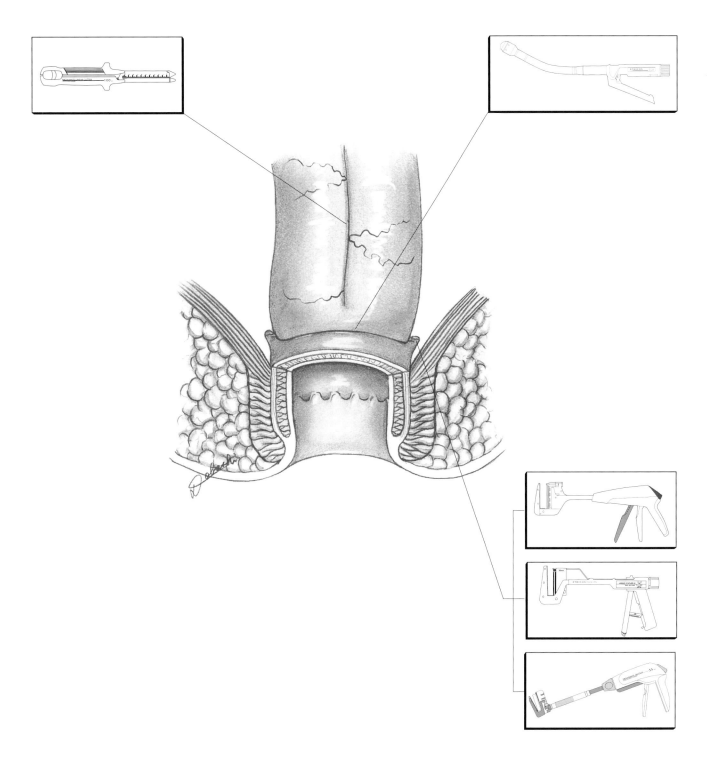

The diagram illustrates one of various possibilities for the construction of a reservoir
following a total colectomy.

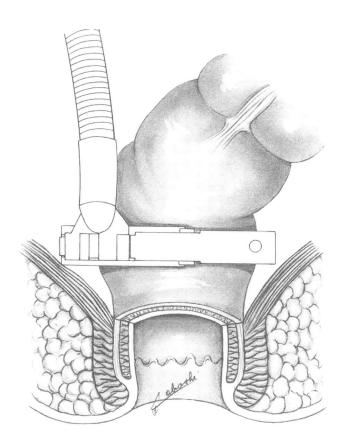

The procedure begins with mobilization of the
colon to be resected using suture ligatures, clips,
or the Harmonic Scalpel. The rectum is closed
with an articulating linear stapler.

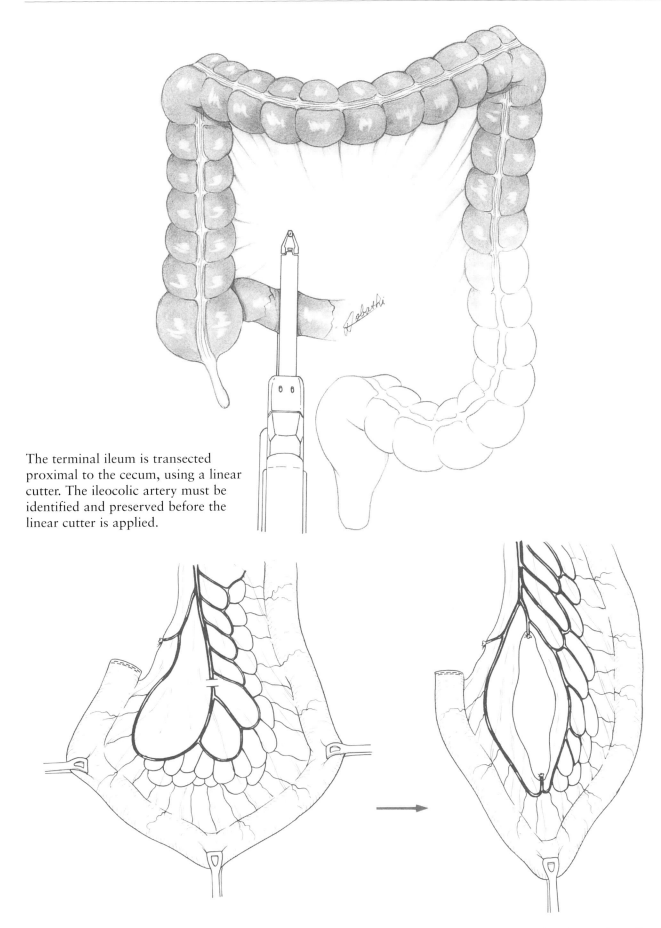

The terminal ileum is transected proximal to the cecum, using a linear cutter. The ileocolic artery must be identified and preserved before the linear cutter is applied.

The loops of ileum are mobilized with suture ligatures, clips, or the Harmonic Scalpel in order to create a mesenteric window for posterior construction of the J-pouch. Adequate length must be obtained to allow tension-free delivery of the ileum into the pelvis for construction of the J-pouch.

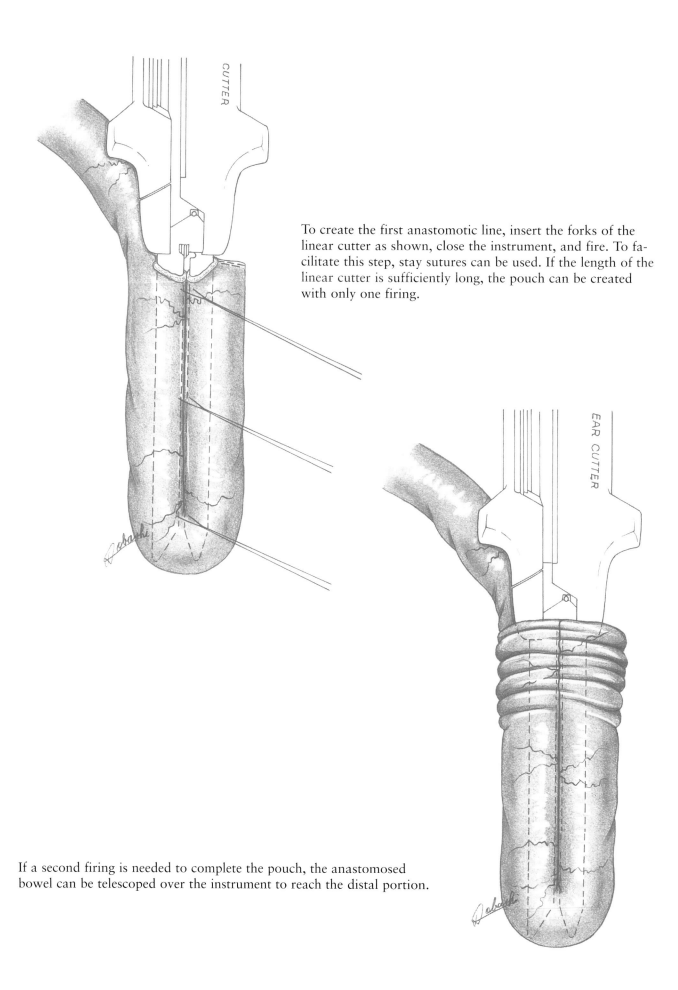

CUTTER

To create the first anastomotic line, insert the forks of the linear cutter as shown, close the instrument, and fire. To facilitate this step, stay sutures can be used. If the length of the linear cutter is sufficiently long, the pouch can be created with only one firing.

EAR CUTTER

If a second firing is needed to complete the pouch, the anastomosed bowel can be telescoped over the instrument to reach the distal portion.

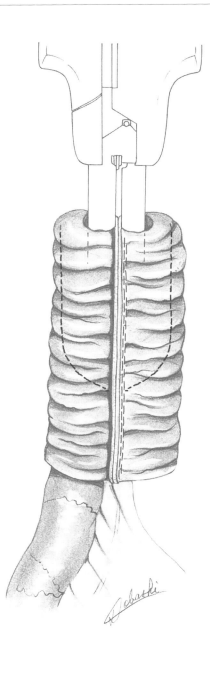

To facilitate eversion of the pouch, leave the linear cutter closed and in place. Once it is everted, check the pouch for hemostasis.

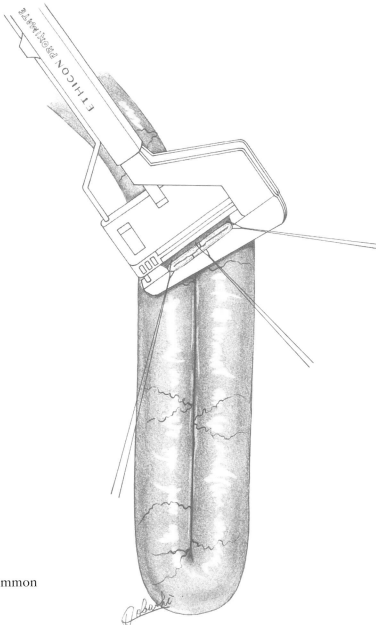

Following construction of the J-pouch, the common opening is closed with a linear stapler.

A purse-string suture is placed in the distal
portion of the pouch, and the anvil of the
circular stapler is inserted into the J-pouch lumen,
through an enterotomy made in the center of
the purse-string. The purse-string suture is tied
around the anvil rod. The circular stapler is
inserted transanally, and the trocar is extended to
pierce the wall of the distal stump. The anvil is
attached to the integral trocar, and the circular
stapler is closed and fired, creating the side-to-end
anastomosis. After the circular stapler is withdrawn, the tissue donuts are examined for completeness. The donuts should be intact and
include all tissue layers. If the donuts are not
complete, the anastomosis should be carefully
checked for leakage and appropriate repairs
made.

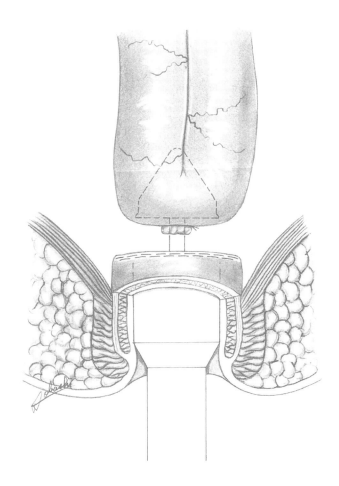

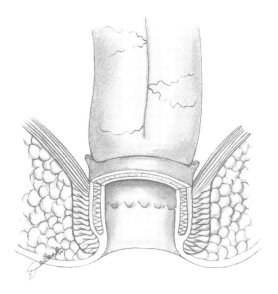

End result.

Colectomy: J-Pouch (2)

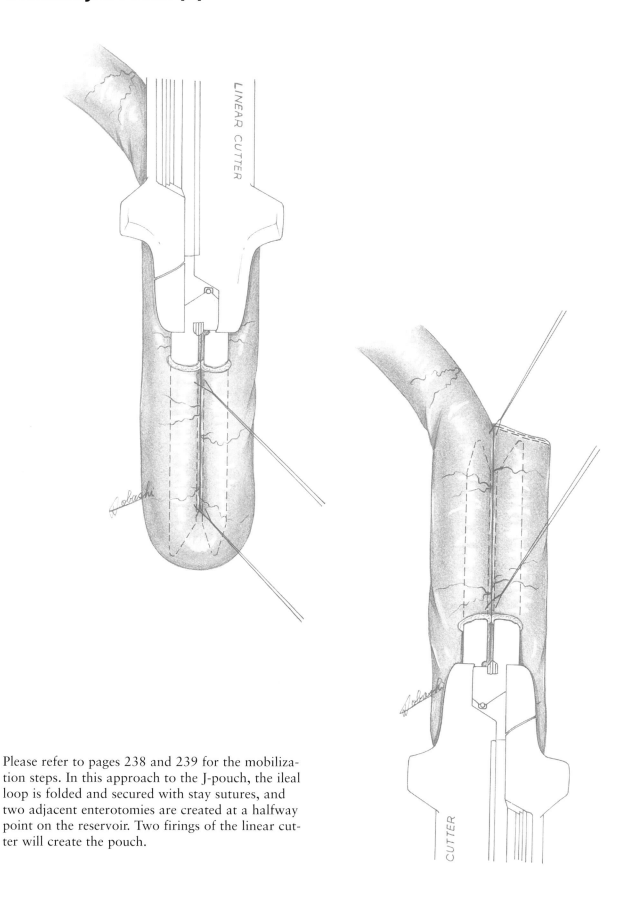

Please refer to pages 238 and 239 for the mobilization steps. In this approach to the J-pouch, the ileal loop is folded and secured with stay sutures, and two adjacent enterotomies are created at a halfway point on the reservoir. Two firings of the linear cutter will create the pouch.

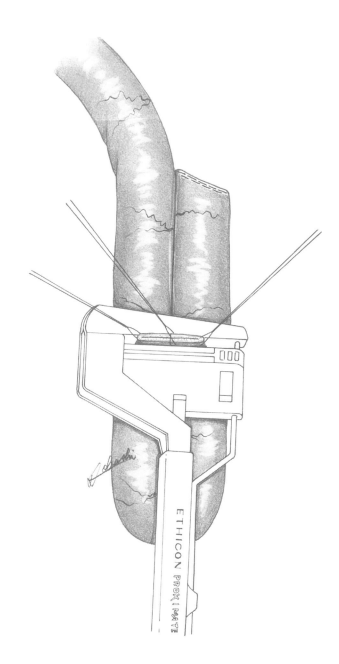

A linear stapler and stay sutures are used to
close the common ileal opening.

Colectomy: J-Pouch (3)

Please refer to pages 238 and 239 for the mobilizaton steps. After the ileal loop has been folded and secured with stay sutures, a distal ileotomy is created to allow the insertion of the linear cutter for the side-to-side anastomosis. If the linear cutter is long enough, this step can be accomplished with only one firing. The distal ileotomy should be of the appropriate size, to allow insertion of the anvil of the circular stapler after creation of the pouch.

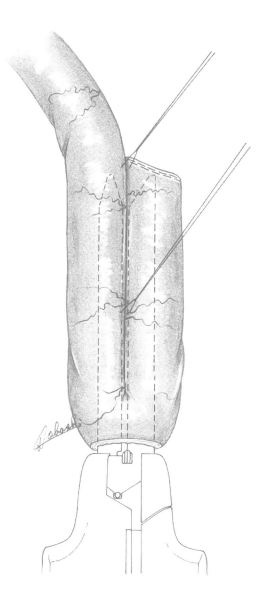

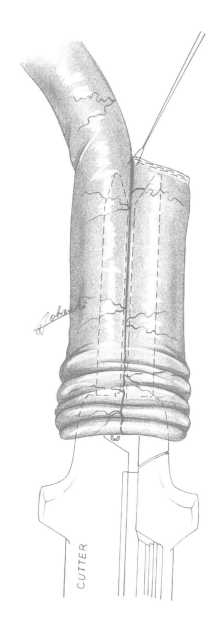

CUTTER

If a second firing is needed to complete the pouch, the anastomosed bowel can be telescoped over the instrument in order to gain access to the distal portion. A purse-string suture is placed in the distal portion of the pouch circumscribing the common opening.
The anvil of the circular stapler is introduced into the J-pouch lumen through the common opening, and the purse-string suture is tied around the anvil center rod. The circular stapler is then inserted transanally, and the trocar is extended to pierce the wall of the distal stump. The anvil is attached to the integral trocar, and the circular stapler is closed and fired, creating the end-to-side anastomosis. After the circular stapler is withdrawn, the tissue donuts are examined for completeness. The donuts should be intact and include all tissue layers. If the donuts are not complete, the anastomosis should be carefully checked for leakage and appropriate repairs made.

Colectomy: W-Pouch

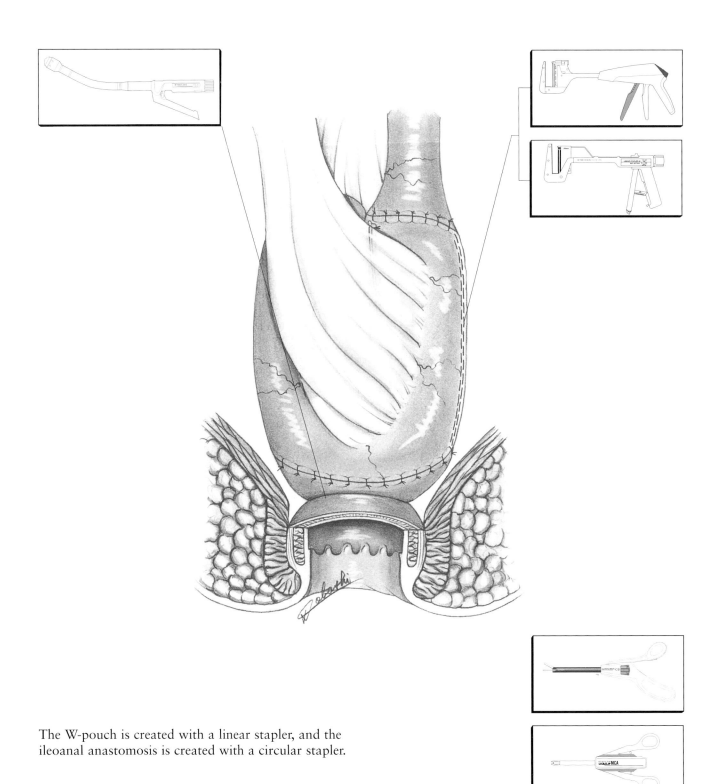

The W-pouch is created with a linear stapler, and the
ileoanal anastomosis is created with a circular stapler.

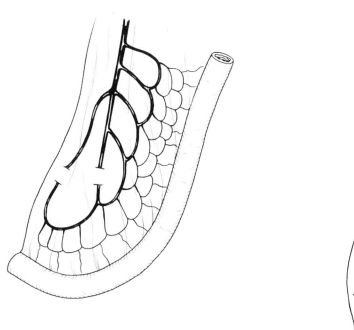 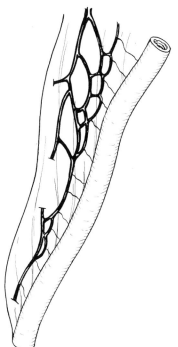

The procedure begins with mobilization of the terminal ileum with suture ligatures, clips, or the Harmonic Scalpel. Approximately 50 cm of bowel is required to perform a W-pouch.

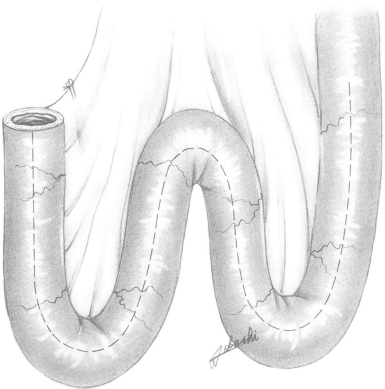

A longitudinal incision is made on the antimesenteric edge of the mobilized ileal loop. The ileum is opened and formed into a W shape.

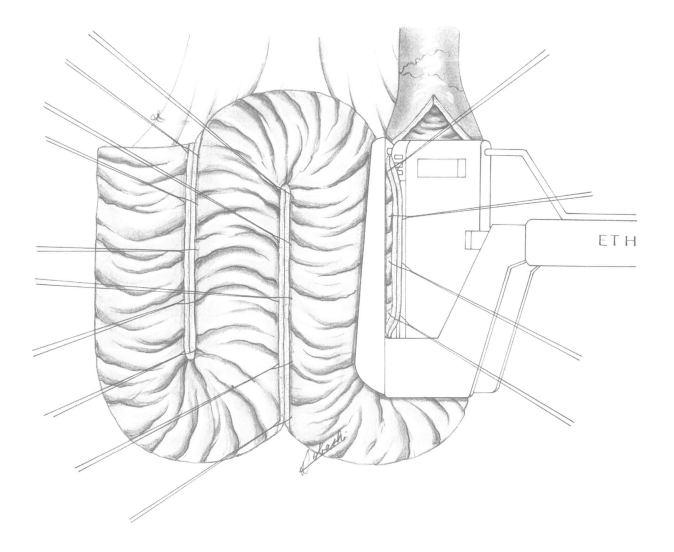

After the W is formed, its shape is maintained with stay sutures. To create the pouch, the approximated edges are stapled with three applications of the linear stapler. Excess tissue, including the stay sutures, is transected along the cutting guide of the stapler.

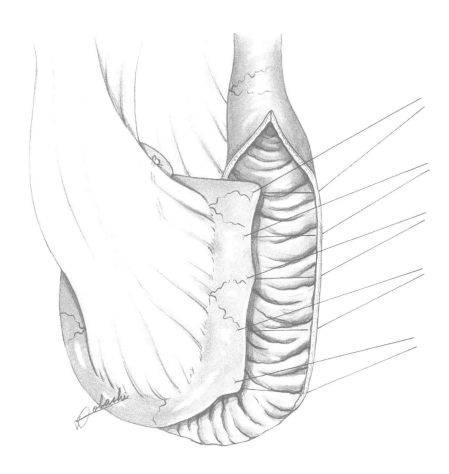

The pouch is closed by approximating the right and left borders with sutures. This can be facilitated with a linear stapler.

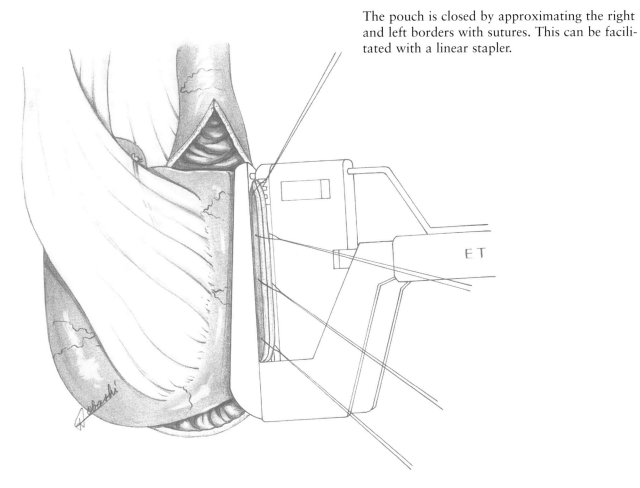

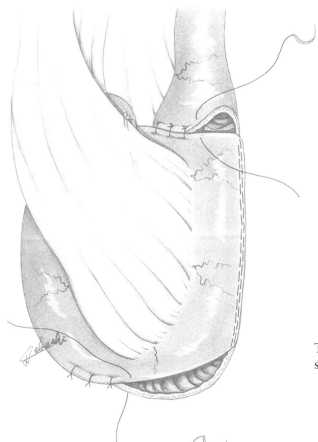

The W-pouch closure is completed with simple sutures.

A purse-string suture is placed in the distal portion of the pouch. An enterotomy is made in the pouch in the center of the area circumscribed by the purse-string suture. The anvil of the circular stapler is inserted into the W-pouch lumen, and the purse-string suture is tied around the anvil's center rod. The circular stapler is then inserted transanally, and the trocar is extended to pierce the wall of the distal stump. The anvil is attached to the integral trocar, and the circular stapler is closed and fired, creating the side-to-end anastomosis. After the circular stapler is withdrawn, the tissue donuts are examined for completeness. The donuts should be intact and include all tissue layers. If the donuts are not complete, the anastomosis should be carefully checked for leakage and appropriate repairs made.

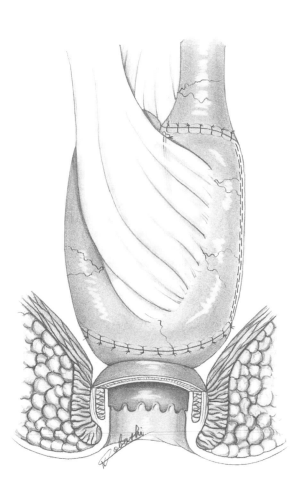

Results of the W-pouch after an ileoanal anastomosis with the circular stapler.

Procedure for Prolapse and Hemorrhoids – PPH

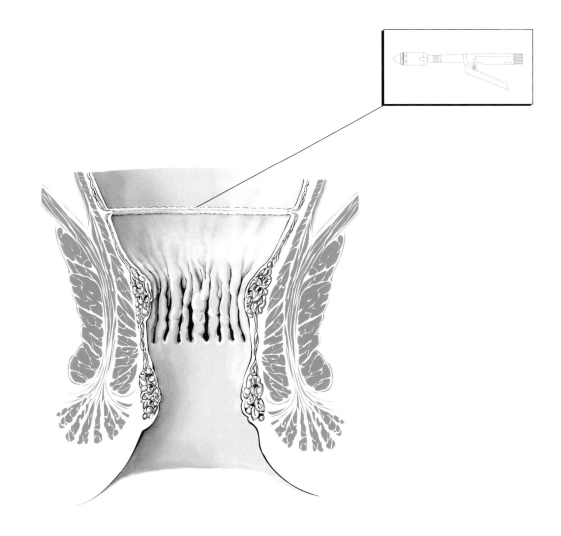

This procedure is for the treatment of hemorrhoidal disease through the circular excision of a band of prolapsed mucosa proximal to the dentate line (anal lifting). A kit has been specifically designed for this procedure. It contains a 33-mm short-shaft circular stapler, a circular anal dilator, a purse-string suture anoscope, and a suture threader.

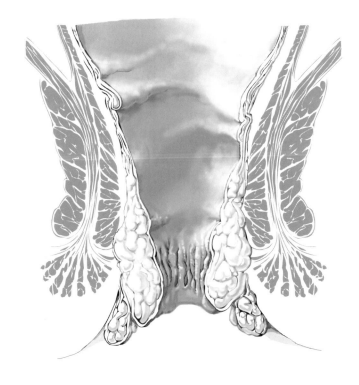

The typical morphological situation of the hemorrhoidal and mucous prolapse is caused by weakening and breakage of the supporting muscular and connective fibers. Prolapse implies the distal dislocation of the internal hemorrhoidal cushions, pushing the external hemorrhoidal sacks in an outward and lateral direction, thus causing the sacks to protrude. The upper hemorrhoidal vessels extend, while the middle and lower hemorrhoidal vessels are subject to the formation of "kinks." The hemorrhoidal volume may remain normal or swell, owing to phlebostasis. It may also regress toward atrophy. In 4th degree prolapse, the dentate line is positioned almost outside the anal canal, and the rectal mucous membrane permanently occupies the muscular anal canal.

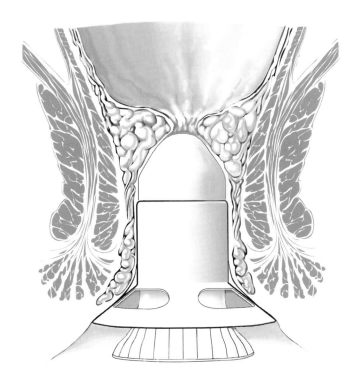

Introduction of the circular anal dilator causes the reduction of the prolapse of anoderm and parts of the anal mucous membrane. To hold the circular anal dilator in place optimally, it should be sutured to the anoderm at the four cardinal points. After the obturator is removed, the prolapsed mucous membrane falls into the lumen of the dilator. The transparency of the device allows viewing of the dentate line.

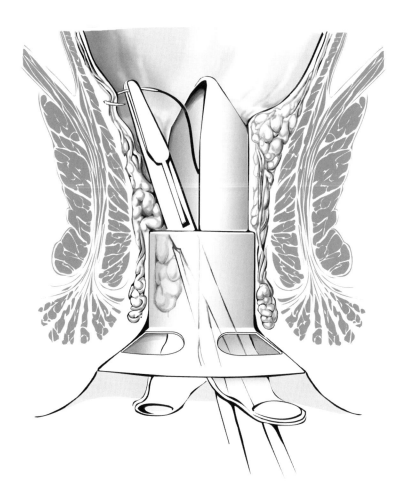

The purse-string suture anoscope is introduced through the anal dilator.
This instrument will move the mucous prolapse along the rectal walls along a
270° circumference. The mucous membrane, which protrudes through
the window of the purse-string suture anoscope, can easily be contained in a
monofilament suture which only includes the mucous membrane. This suture has
to be placed at least 5 cm proximal to the dentate line, since it is necessary to
increase the distance in proportion to the degree of the prolapse. Rotating the
purse-string suture anoscope enables the placement of a purse-string suture
around the entire anal circumference. In the case of asymmetric prolapse, it is
possible to carry out two "half purse-strings," their distance being established
according to need.

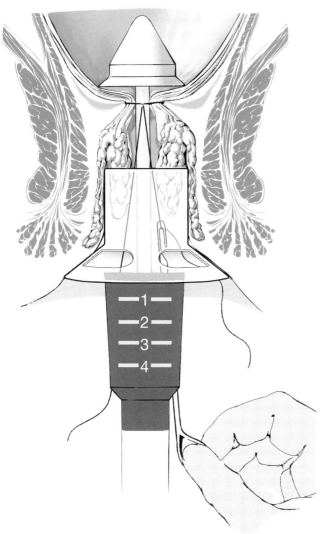

The short-shaft circular stapler is opened to its maximum position. Its head is introduced and positioned proximal to the purse-string, which is then tied with a closing knot. With the help of the suture threader, the ends of the threads are pulled through the lateral holes of the stapler.

The ends of the threads are knotted externally or fixed using forceps. The entire casing or staple housing of the circular stapler is introduced to the anal canal. During the introduction, it is advisable to partially tighten the stapler.

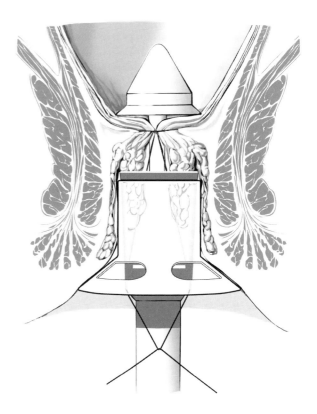

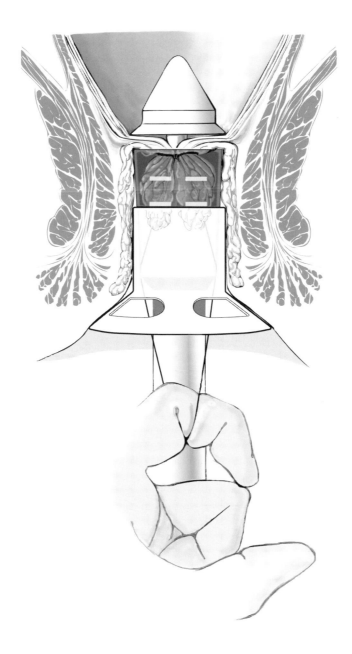

With moderate traction on the purse-string suture, a simple maneuver causes
the prolapsed mucous membrane to be drawn into the casing. Tightening of the
circular stapler is completed, and the stapling of the prolapse is carried out.
Allowing the instrument to remain closed in this position for 20 seconds before
and after firing acts as a tamponade and may enhance hemostasis. The stapler
is then partially opened, rotated 90° in both directions, and withdrawn.
The tissue specimens (donuts) are removed from the stapler. The staple line
is then examined using the purse-string suture anoscope, which enables the
addition of stitches, if needed.

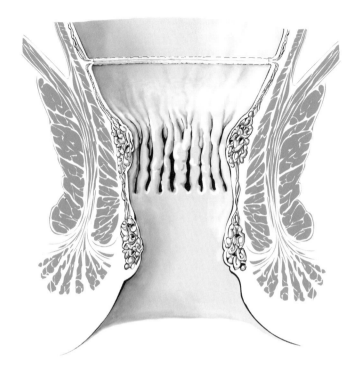

This technique and the instrument kit ensure correct placement of the mucosomucosal anastomosis at least 2 cm proximal to the dentate line. The circular anal dilator preserves the unstriated internal sphincter and permits atraumatic placement of a purse-string suture. The purse-string suture anoscope assists the measurement of the distance between the purse-string suture and the dentate line, and simplifies its placement. The circular stapler is very easy to handle, and enables simultaneous resection of larger rectal prolapses. The possibility of standardizing the prolapse resection, graduating the traction of the threads and the height of the purse-string, is an important improvement to the technique.

8 Gynecological Surgery

Salpingectomy

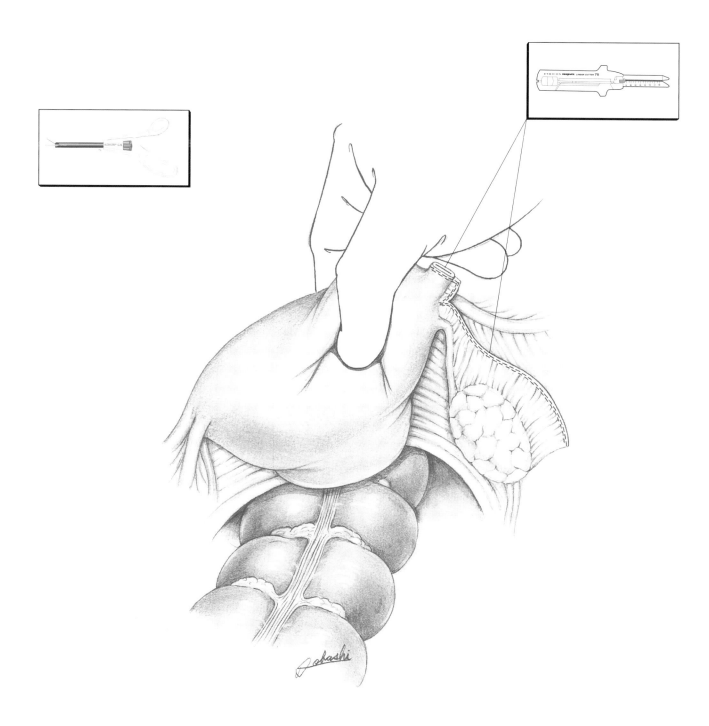

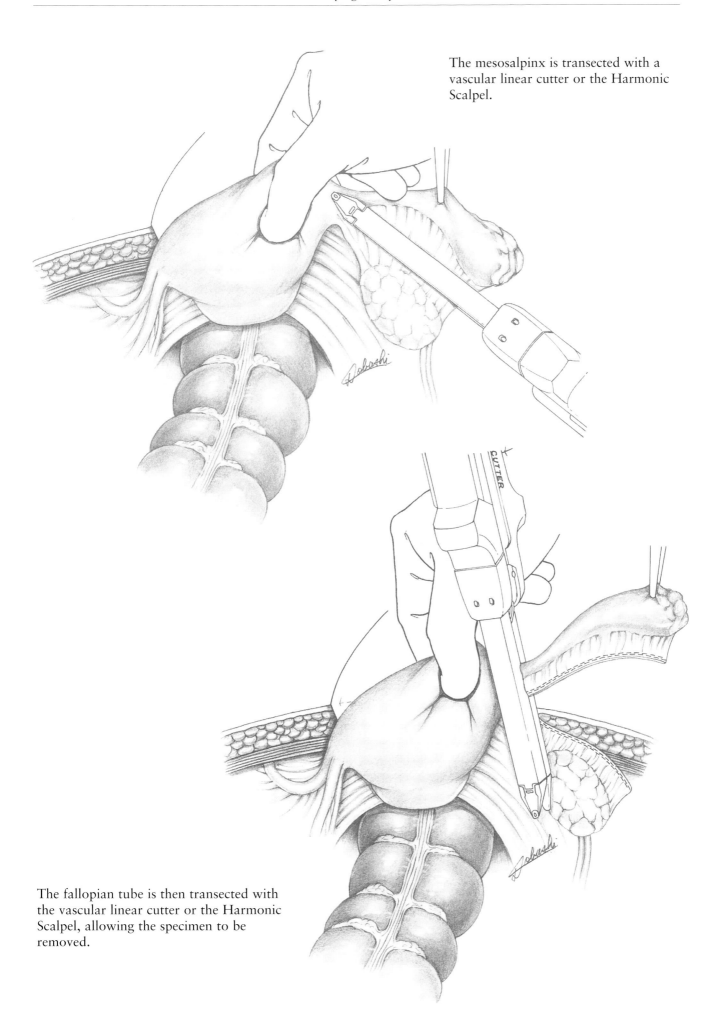

The mesosalpinx is transected with a vascular linear cutter or the Harmonic Scalpel.

The fallopian tube is then transected with the vascular linear cutter or the Harmonic Scalpel, allowing the specimen to be removed.

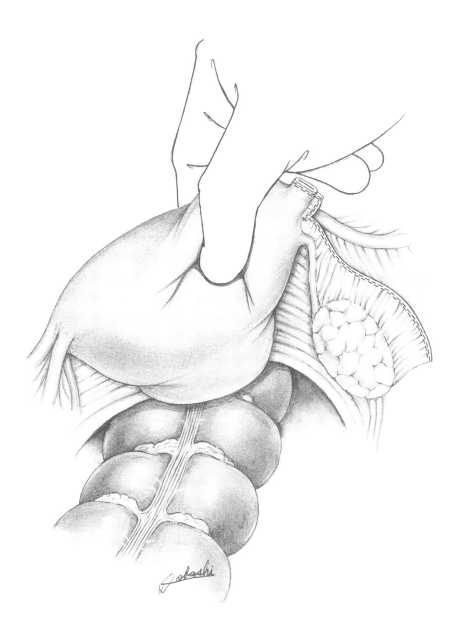

The staple lines are examined for hemostasis and
proper staple closure.

Salpingo-Oophorectomy

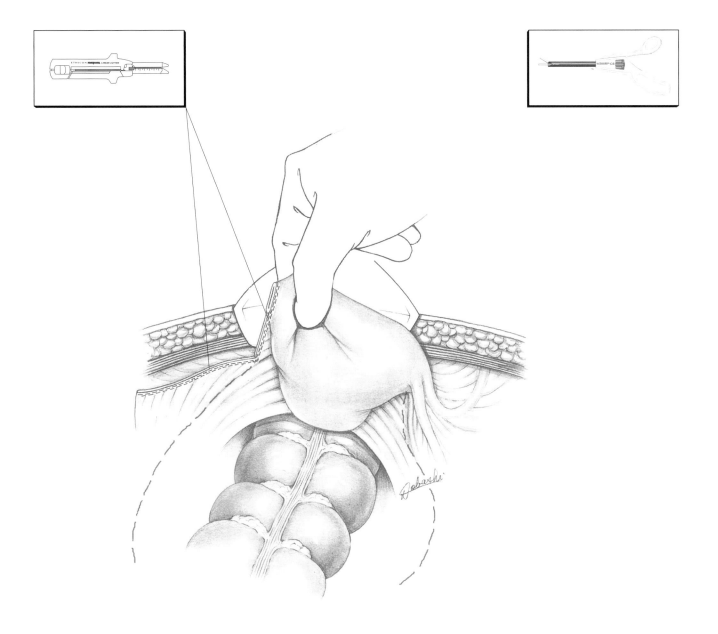

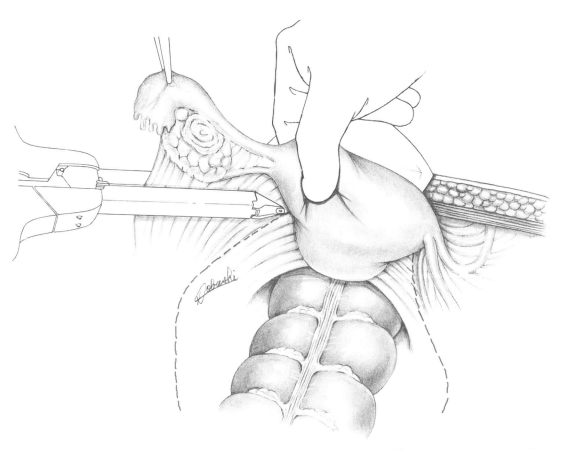

The mesometrium and the infundibulopelvic ligament are transected with the vascular linear cutter or the Harmonic Scalpel.

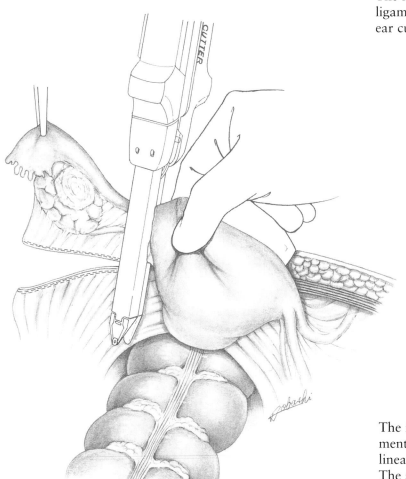

The fallopian tube and utero-ovarian ligament are then transected with the vascular linear cutter or the Harmonic Scalpel. The specimen is removed.

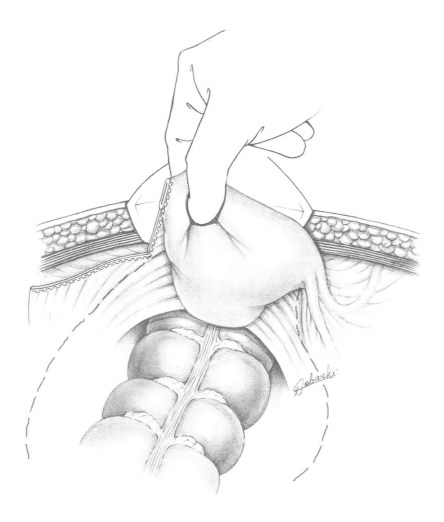

The staple lines are examined for hemostasis and
proper staple closure.

Total Hysterectomy without BSO

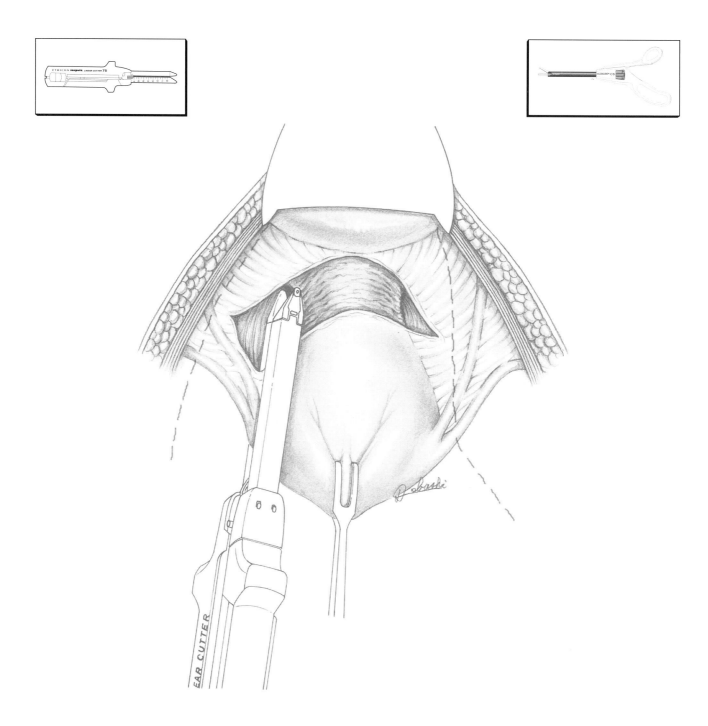

Identify and locate the ureters. The peritoneum is incised transversely in the vesicouterine space to establish a plane between the bladder anteriorly and the uterus posteriorly. One of the broad ligaments is transected using a vascular linear cutter or the Harmonic Scalpel. Examine the staple lines for hemostasis and proper staple closure.

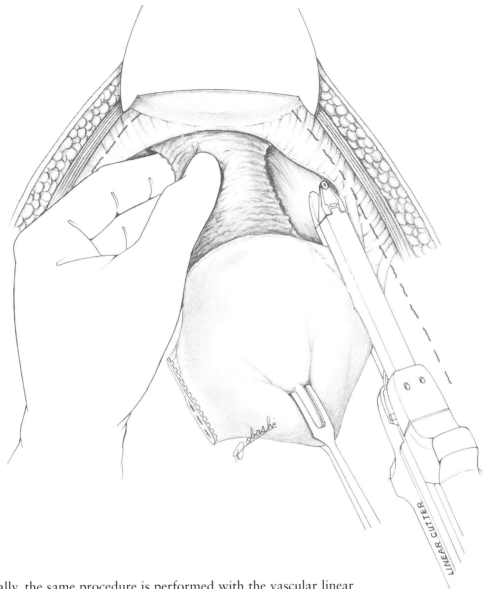

Contralaterally, the same procedure is performed with the vascular linear cutter or the Harmonic Scalpel. The uterine vessels are dissected, ligated, and transected. The cardinal ligaments, which are in close proximity to the uterine arteries, are ligated and divided. This will allow the lateral fornices to be visualized. The uterosacral ligaments are dissected, ligated, and transected. This will allow the posterior fornix to be visualized.

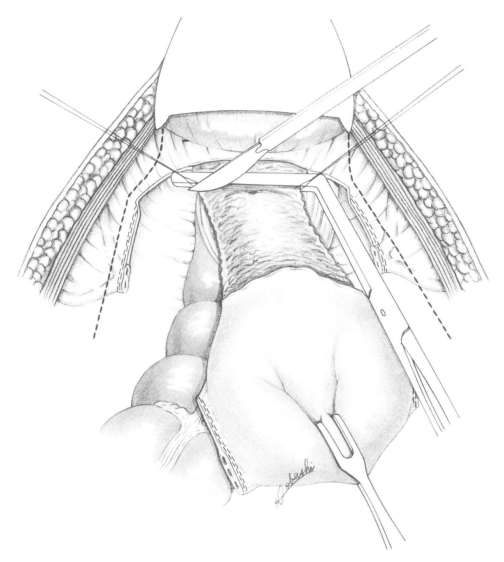

The fornices are incised close to their attachment to the cervix.
The hysterectomy is completed by placing a clamp distal to the
uterine cervix, which is then resected with a scalpel. The vaginal
cuff is closed.

9 Urological Surgery

Following a cystectomy, urine must be drained externally. In principle we distinguish between two approaches for facilitating this drainage: "incontinent" and "continent" urination.

"Incontinent" Urination

If there is no possibility of creating a continent pouch, urine must be drained into an adhesive bag.

Different methods can be used for this kind of procedure:

Ureteral Skin Fistula (Cutaneous Ureterostomy)

One or both ureters are sewn directly into the skin. If possible, a ureteroureterostomy is performed, so only one collecting bag is necessary.

Renal Fistula (Nephrostomy)

One ureter is anastomosed to the contralateral renal pelvis. The urine is drained from this renal pelvis via a catheter connected to an exterior collecting bag.

Ileal conduit

A segment of small intestine is isolated, leaving the vascular supply intact. One end of this segment is sewn into the skin, as performed in an ileostomy, while the other end of the segment is closed. The ureters are then implanted into the conduit. This procedure can also be performed with a segment of the colon (colonic conduit).

The following is an example of a procedure using an ileal conduit:

Ileal Conduit – Bricker Technique

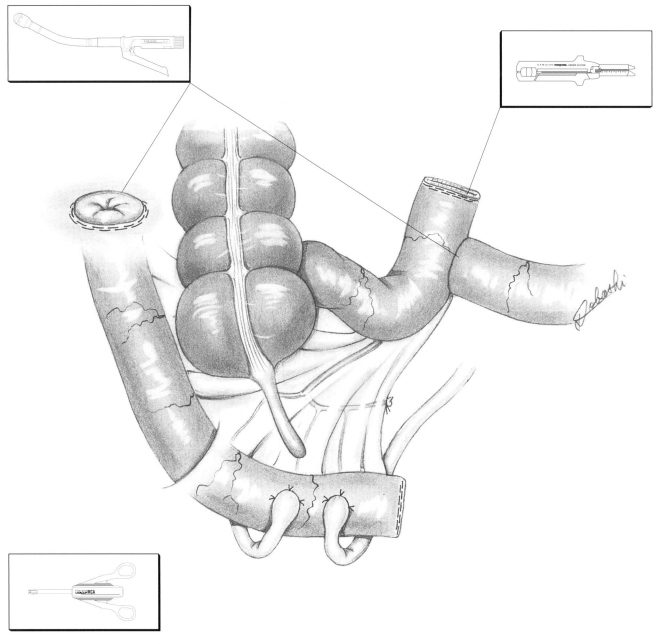

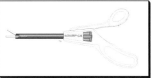

The ileal conduit was developed by Dr. Bricker in 1950 and has been the leading incontinent technique for urinary drainage. Today, however, continent techniques for urinary drainage are preferred. Long-term results of this new type of operation remain unknown to a great extent, so some urologists still use the Bricker operation, which has been tested for over 40 years.

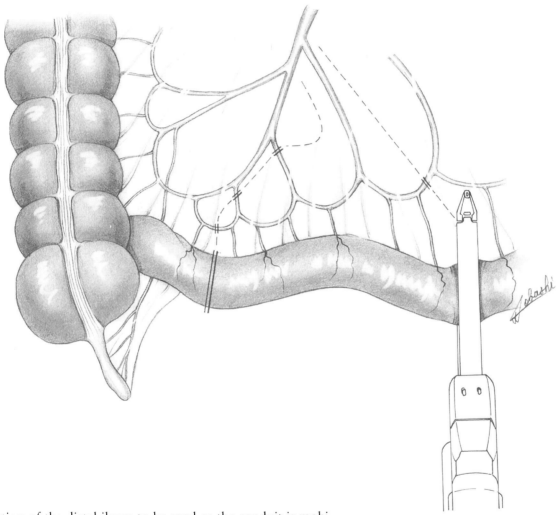

The portion of the distal ileum to be used as the conduit is mobilized using suture ligatures, clips, or the Harmonic Scalpel.
The distal ileal segment is isolated by firing the linear cutter twice.

A variety of techniques may be used to recreate intestinal continuity.
The diagram on pages 268 and 270 depict a completed end-to-side ileoileostomy.
Below is a diagram and description of a side-to-end ileoileostomy.

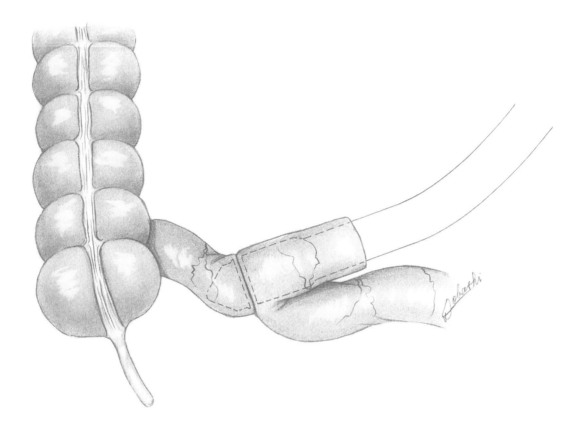

At the proximal end of the distal segment, a purse-string suture is placed and the
staple line is resected. The anvil of the circular stapler is inserted into the lumen
of the proximal end of the distal segment, and the purse-string suture is tied
around the anvil center rod. The staple line at the distal end of the proximal segment is resected to allow for the insertion of the circular stapler. The circular stapler is inserted into the lumen of the proximal segment. The ileal wall is pierced
by the integral trocar on the antimesenteric border. The anvil is attached to the
integral trocar tip, and the circular stapler is closed and fired, creating the side-
to-end ileoileostomy. After the circular stapler is withdrawn, the tissue donuts are
examined for completeness. The donuts should be intact and include all tissue
layers. If the donuts are not complete, the anastomosis should be carefully
checked for leakage and appropriate repairs made. The remaining ileotomy,
which is the distal end of the proximal segment, is closed with a linear cutter
approximately 3 cm from the anastomosis.

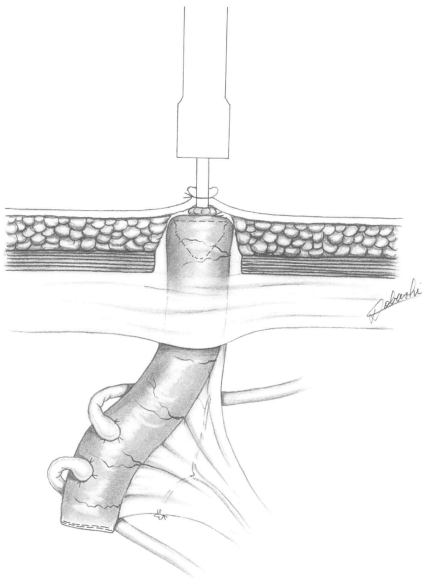

Both ureters are anastomosed to the antimesenteric side of the ileal conduit. Position the ileal conduit, and place a purse-string suture on the segment to be exteriorized. The anvil of the circular stapler is inserted into the ileal lumen, and the purse-string is tied. Another purse-string suture is placed at the skin level. The cutaneous purse-string suture is also tied around the shaft of the anvil. The anvil is attached to the integral trocar, and the circular stapler is closed and fired, creating the end-to-end ileo-cutaneous anastomosis. After the circular stapler is withdrawn, the tissue donuts are examined for completeness. The donuts should be intact and include all tissue layers. If the donuts are not complete, the anastomosis should be carefully checked for leakage and appropriate repairs made.

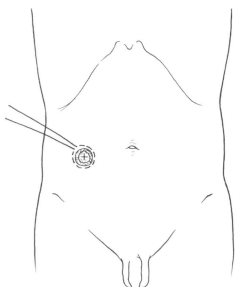

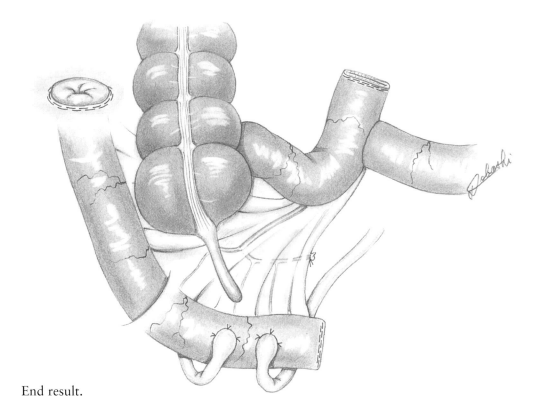

End result.

"Continent" Urination

To perform procedures for continent urination in males, the patient must have a healthy urethra, as well as ureters with healthy distal ends. If this is not the case, then continent stomata or natural orifices must be used in order to achieve continence.

Ureterosigmoidostomy

The ureters are anastomosed to the sigmoid colon. Urine and stools are then excreted together. When a large reservoir is desired, the Mainz Pouch II techniqued is used (Figure below).

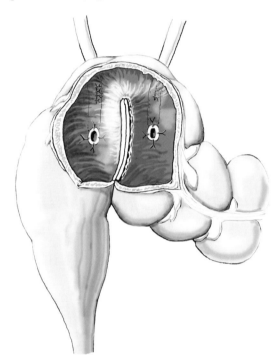
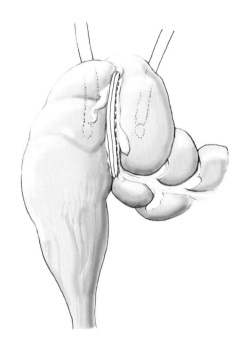

Ileal Neobladder

The ureters can be inserted into a neobladder created with small intestine. A 60- to 70-cm segment of small intestine is mobilized and isolated in order to create a replacement bladder. Both ureters are anastomosed at the upper part of the new bladder to avoid urine reflux. The urethra is sewn to the lower part of the intestinal bladder. The ileal neobladder permits normal voiding in most cases.

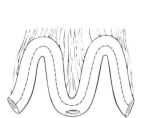
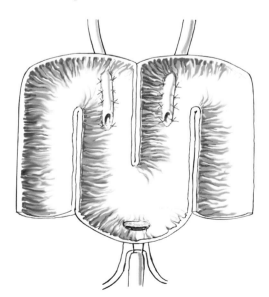
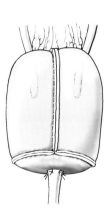

Intestinal Pouch with a Catheterizible Stoma

A reservoir is created from a small or large intestinal segment, or a combination of the two, to which the ureters are connected. The stoma of the reservoir is exteriorized at a cosmetically favorable place, e.g., in the region of the umbilicus, using an intestinal segment or the appendix. Since there is no sphincter, the outlet is narrowed surgically to the extent of making the reservoir leak-proof. The patient empties the reservoir by using a catheter (three to four times every day, once during the night).

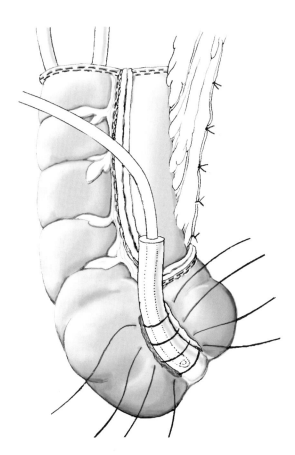

Following are examples of procedures using this type of approach:

Ileal Reservoir – Urological Kock Pouch

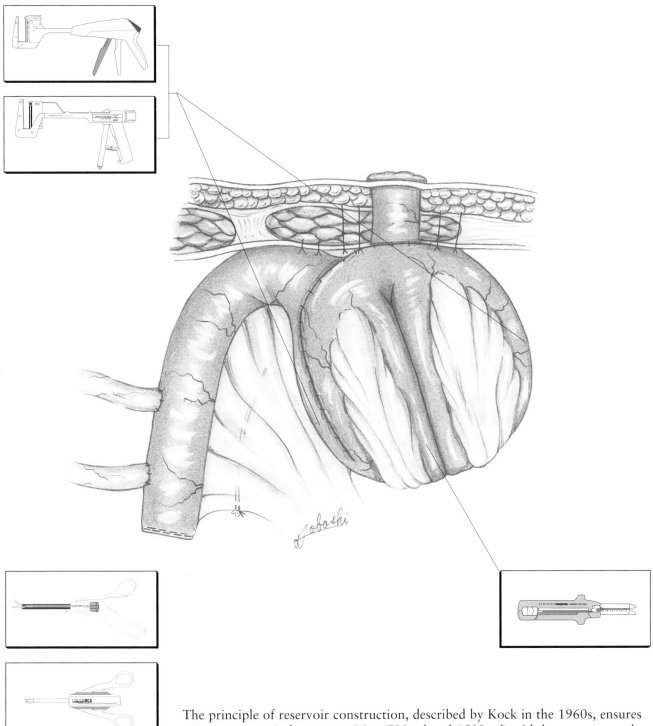

The principle of reservoir construction, described by Kock in the 1960s, ensures urinary storage in large quantities (700 ml and 1500 ml) with low pressure values. The success of the operation depends on the construction and maintenance of the nipple valve mechanism. Complications occur in over 30% of cases, and over 18% of the patients submit to reoperation in order to restore continence. Long-term observations indicate the patients accept this procedure, but this technique is seldom used because of the high complication rate.

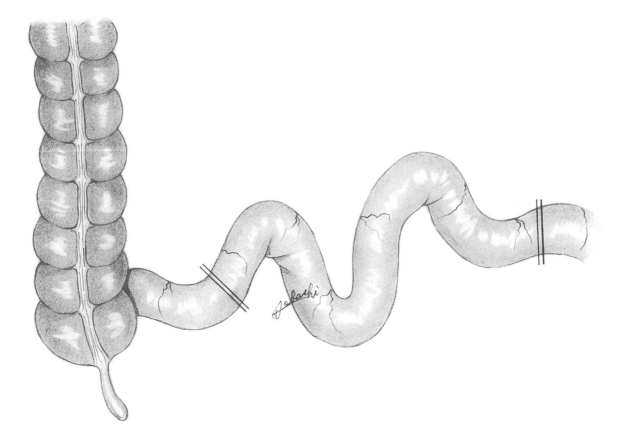

A 30-cm loop of the terminal ileum is mobilized using suture ligatures, clips, or the Harmonic Scalpel. An isolated ileal segment with preserved blood supply is created with two firings of the linear cutter. The staple lines are examined for hemostasis and proper staple closure.

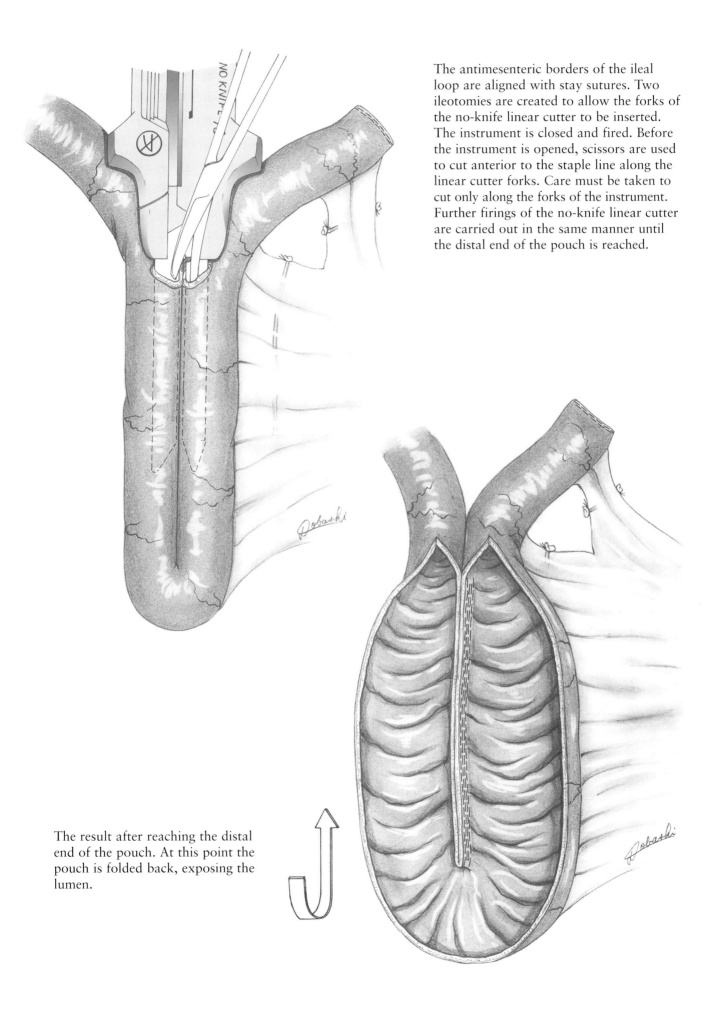

The antimesenteric borders of the ileal loop are aligned with stay sutures. Two ileotomies are created to allow the forks of the no-knife linear cutter to be inserted. The instrument is closed and fired. Before the instrument is opened, scissors are used to cut anterior to the staple line along the linear cutter forks. Care must be taken to cut only along the forks of the instrument. Further firings of the no-knife linear cutter are carried out in the same manner until the distal end of the pouch is reached.

The result after reaching the distal end of the pouch. At this point the pouch is folded back, exposing the lumen.

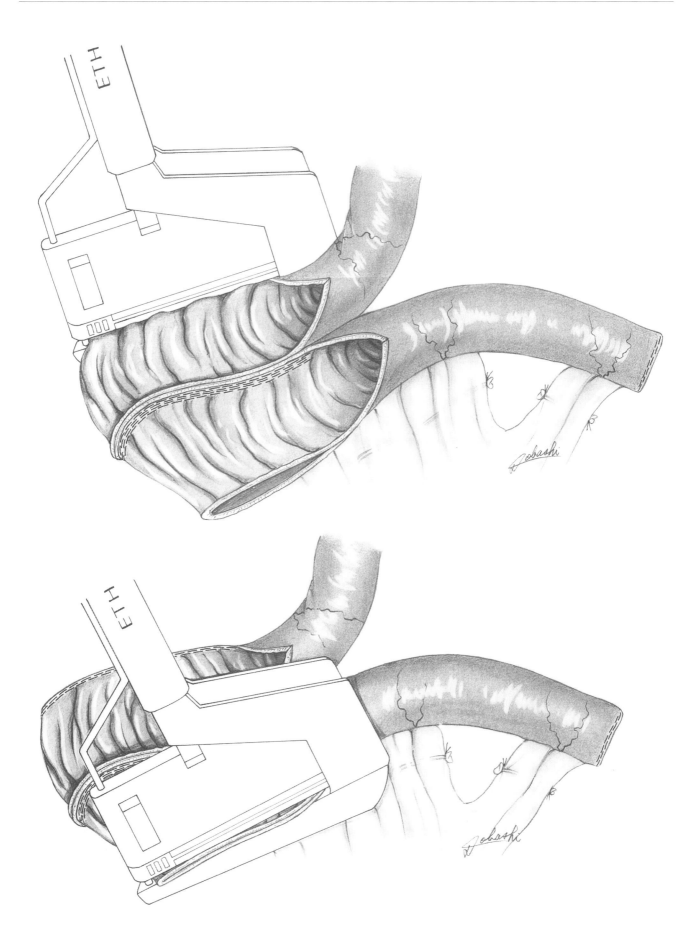

The external edges of the pouch are approximated with a linear stapler.

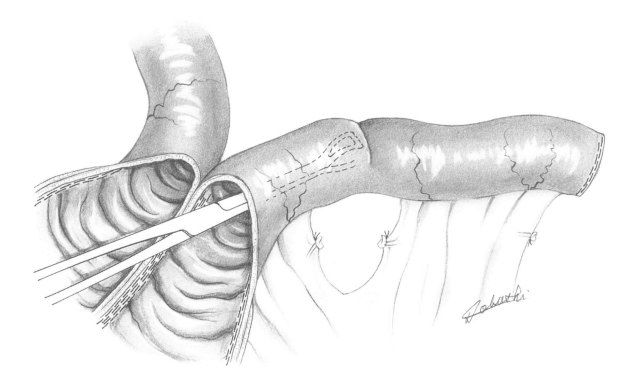

A 10-cm mesenteric window is created in the distal end of the ileal segment to facilitate intussusception. It is preferable to avoid using clips in this area. The ileum is intussuscepted by inserting an atraumatic clamp into the lumen for a distance of approximately 5 cm and grasping the ileal mucosa. The bowel is then pulled back through the lumen until the 5-cm segment is exposed. This maneuver creates a nipple valve.

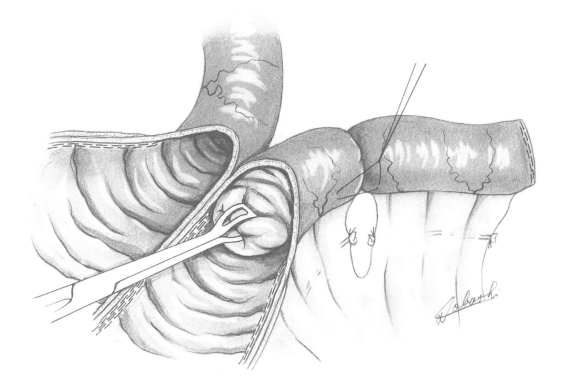

After completing the 5-cm intussusception, stay sutures are placed for fixation.

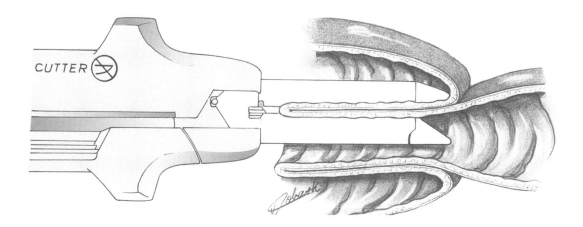

The no-knife linear cutter is fired at the 12, 3, 6, and 9 o'clock positions on the intussusceptum. These four staple lines secure the nipple valve.

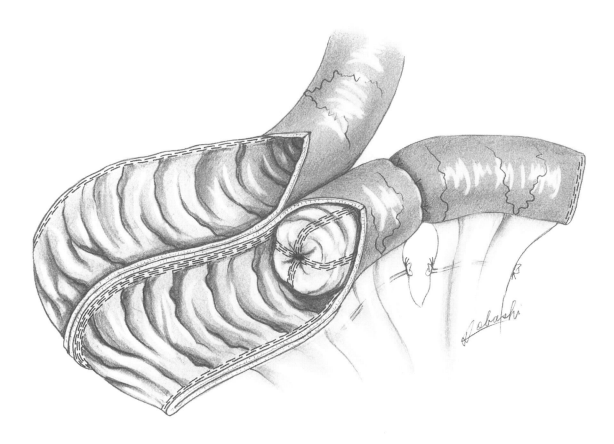

It is critical to examine the staple lines for hemostasis and proper staple closure.

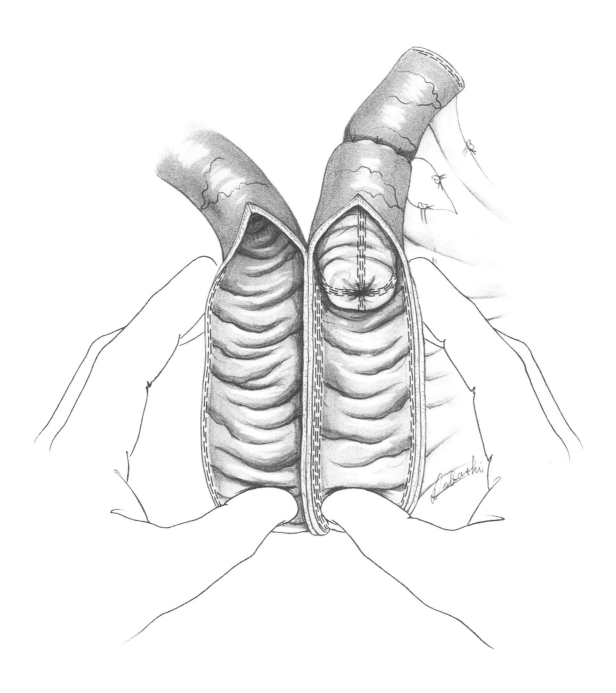

Completed nipple valve.

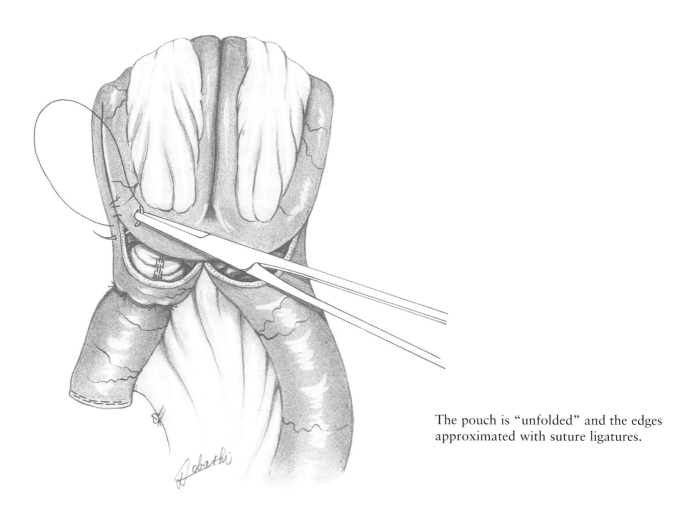

The pouch is "unfolded" and the edges approximated with suture ligatures.

The ureters are anastomosed into the proximal ileal segment. The distal end of the ileal segment, which contains the nipple valve, is exteriorized on the abdominal wall and secured to the skin.

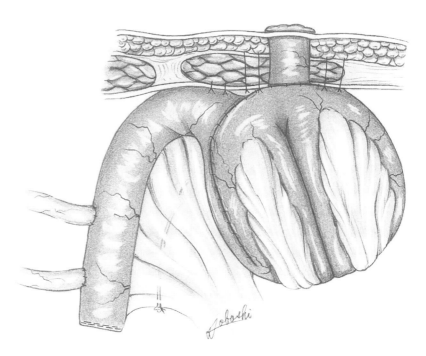

Indiana Pouch

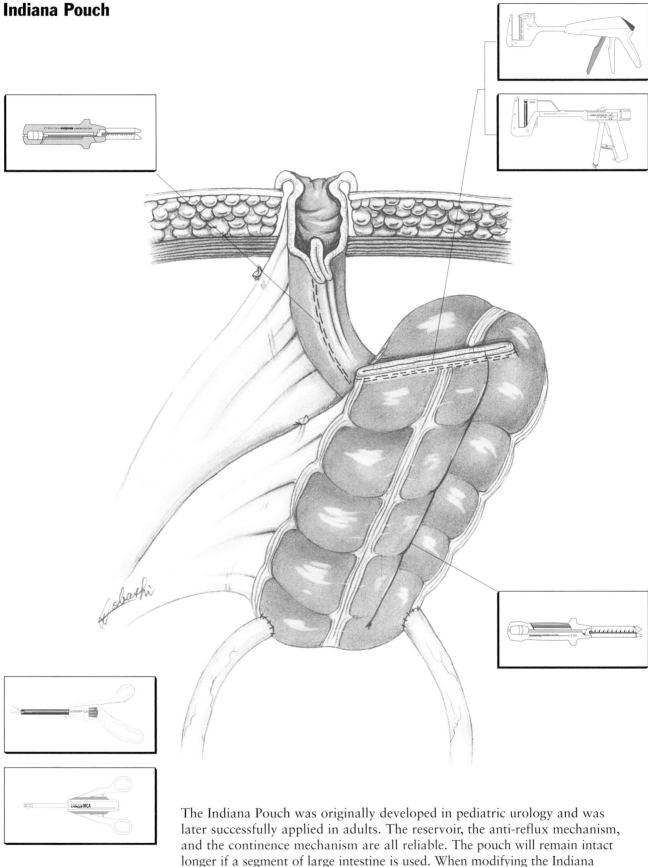

The Indiana Pouch was originally developed in pediatric urology and was later successfully applied in adults. The reservoir, the anti-reflux mechanism, and the continence mechanism are all reliable. The pouch will remain intact longer if a segment of large intestine is used. When modifying the Indiana Pouch, the appendix may be used for urinary drainage to the umbilicus.
The so-called Mainz Pouch I is a variation of the Indiana Pouch principle.

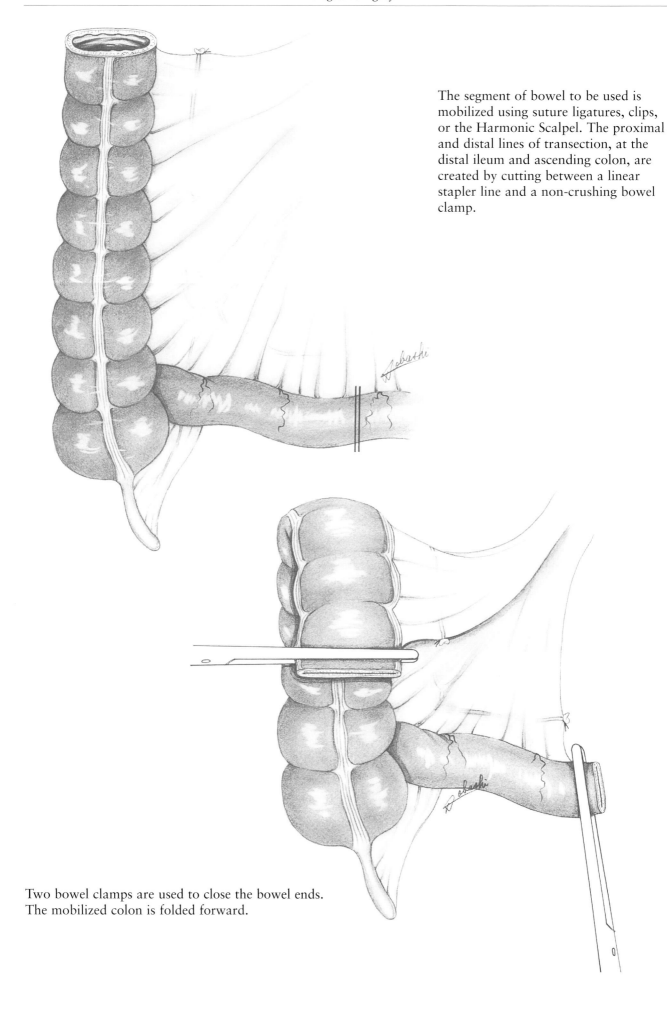

The segment of bowel to be used is mobilized using suture ligatures, clips, or the Harmonic Scalpel. The proximal and distal lines of transection, at the distal ileum and ascending colon, are created by cutting between a linear stapler line and a non-crushing bowel clamp.

Two bowel clamps are used to close the bowel ends. The mobilized colon is folded forward.

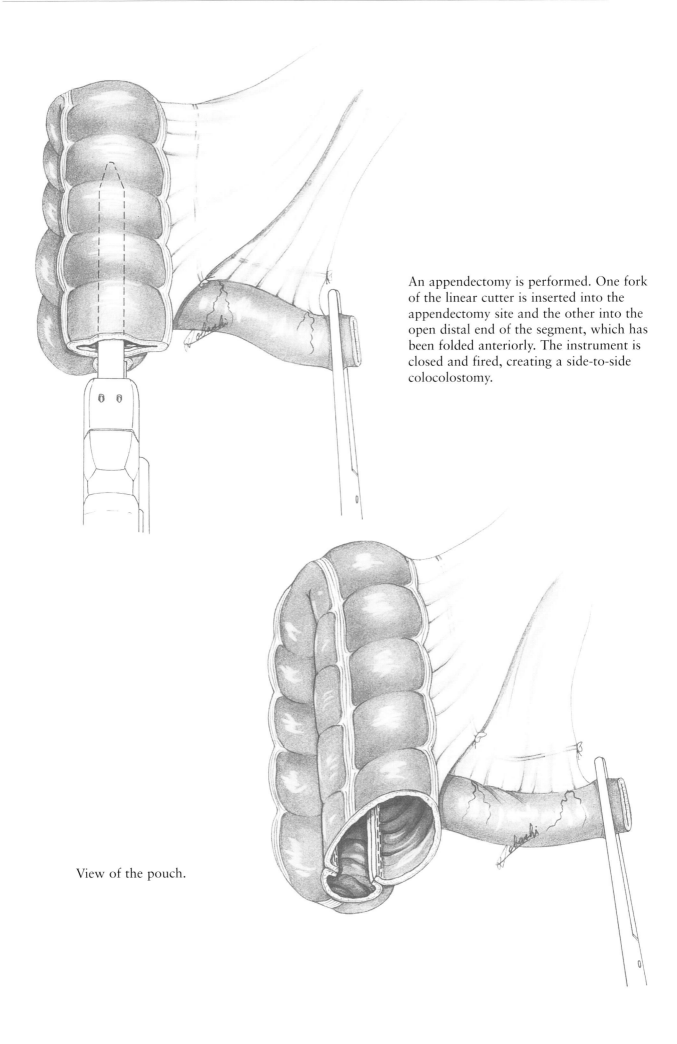

An appendectomy is performed. One fork of the linear cutter is inserted into the appendectomy site and the other into the open distal end of the segment, which has been folded anteriorly. The instrument is closed and fired, creating a side-to-side colocolostomy.

View of the pouch.

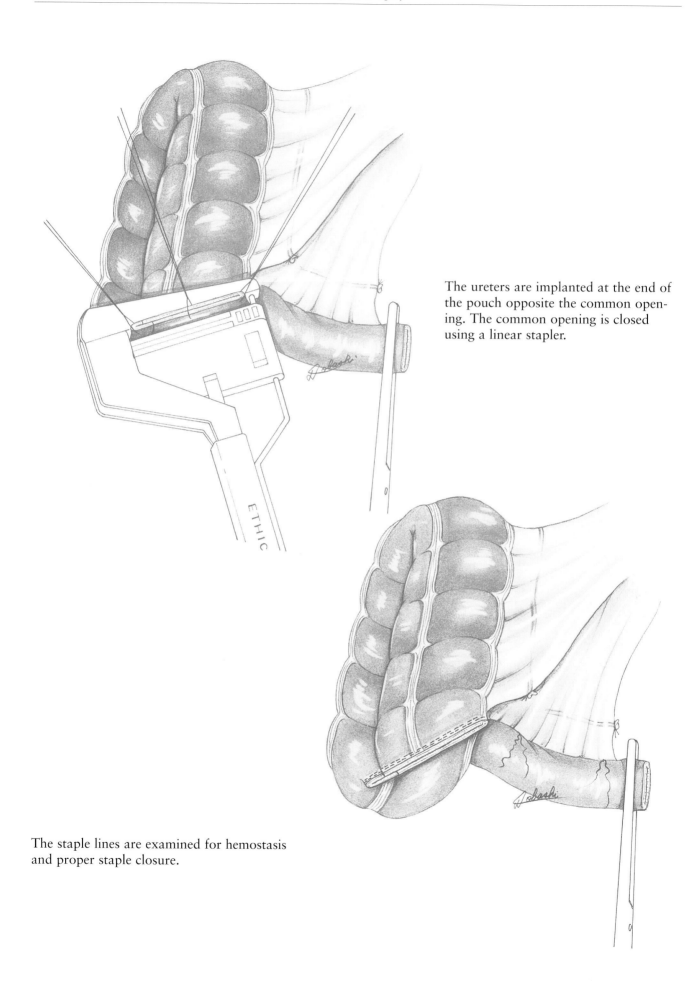

The ureters are implanted at the end of the pouch opposite the common opening. The common opening is closed using a linear stapler.

The staple lines are examined for hemostasis and proper staple closure.

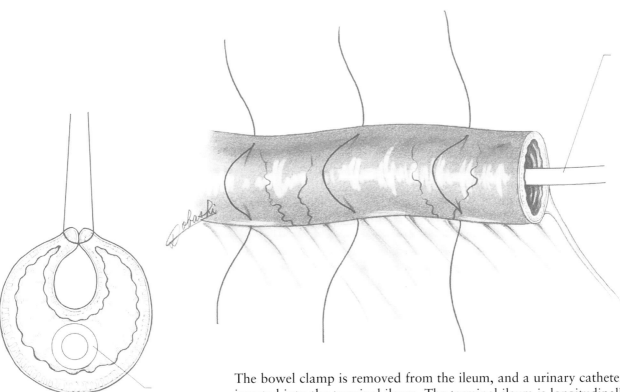

The bowel clamp is removed from the ileum, and a urinary catheter is inserted into the terminal ileum. The terminal ileum is longitudinally folded over the catheter and sutured into position.

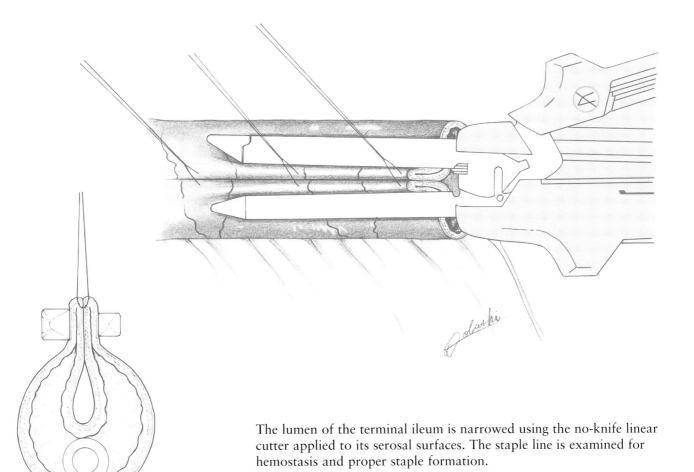

The lumen of the terminal ileum is narrowed using the no-knife linear cutter applied to its serosal surfaces. The staple line is examined for hemostasis and proper staple formation.

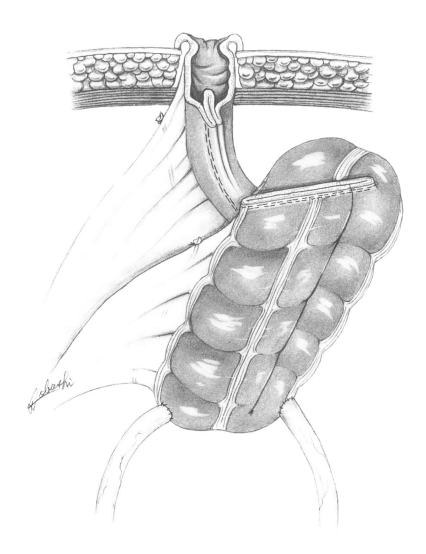

The procedure is completed by exteriorizing the terminal ileum
(ileostomy). The Bauhin valve renders the pouch leak-proof.

Mainz-Pouch I

A modification of the Indiana Pouch is the Mainz Pouch I. In contrast to the
Indiana Pouch, in which continence is achieved by the ileocecal valve in con-
junction with a constriction of the efferent ileal loop, continence in the Mainz
Pouch I is obtained by intussusception of the terminal ileum combined with the
corresponding creation of a nipple. After completion, the nipple is led through
the ileocecal valve and fixed at the cecal portion.

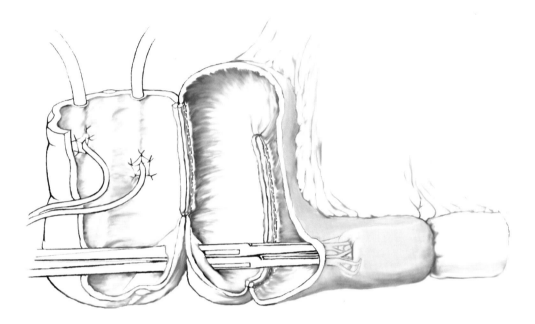

After creating a pouch with part of the proximal ascending colon and the terminal
ileum, a mesenteric window of approximately 10 cm is made at the distal ileum using
the Harmonic Scalpel. To perform the intussusception, two Allis clamps are inserted
through the ileocecal opening into the lumen of the remaining ileum and up to the
middle of the mesenteric window.

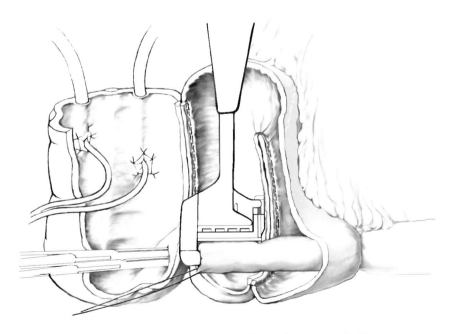

The intussusception is fixed at 3 and 9 o'clock respectively, with two staple lines.
In order to avoid formation of calculi at the top of the nipple, the last three
staples are removed from the cartridge of the linear stapler.

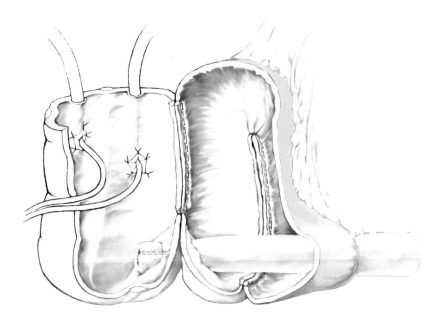

After the nipple has been pulled through the ileocecal valve, it is stapled onto the anterior aspect for fixation.

III

References

Akiyama H, Tsurumaru M, Kawamura T, Ono Y (1981) Principles of surgical treatment for carcinoma of the oesophagus. Ann Surg 194: 438–446

Amaral JF (1993) Laparoscopic application of an ultrasonic activated scalpel. Gastrointest Endosc Clin North Am 3: 381

Amaral JF (1994) Ultrasonic energy in laparoscopic surgery. Surgical Technology International III: 155

Amaral JF (1995) Depth of thermal injury: ultrasonically activated scalpel vs electrosurgery: Surg Endosc 9: 226

Amaral JF (1995) Laparoscopic cholecystectomy in 200 consecutive patients using an ultrasonically activated scalpel. Surg Laparosc Endosc 5: 255

Ata AA, Bellemore TJ, Meisel JA, Arambulo SM (1993) Distal thermal injury from monopolar electrosurgery. Surg Laparosc Endosc 3: 323

Bazan (1989) La chirurgia del tenue e del colon. Le suturatrici meccaniche in chirurgia. Piccin, Padova

Berrisford RG, Page RD, Donnely RJ (1996) Stapler design and strictures at the oesophagogastric anastomosis. J Thorac Cardiovasc Surg 111: 142–146

Berry SM, Ose KJ, Bell RH, Fink AS (1994) Thermal injury of the posterior duodenum during laparoscopic cholecystectomy. Surg Endosc 8: 197

Bell RCW (1996) Can doing more be faster? An ultrasonic scalpel and speed of fundoplication. Surg Endosc 10: 223

Boltri F (1995) Chirurgia dellostomaco con suturatrici meccaniche. Edizioni Minerva Medica, Bologna

Chassin JL (1994) Operative strategy in general surgery, 2nd ed. Springer, New York Heidelberg

Collard JM, Tinton N, Malaise J, Romagnolis R, Otte JB, Kestens PJ (1995) Oesophageal replacement: Gastric tube or whole stomach? Ann Thorac Surg 60: 261–266

Deschamps C (1995) Use of colon and jejunum as possible oesophageal replacements. Chest Surg Clin North Am 5: 555–569

Dewar L, Gelfand G, Finley RJ, Evans K, Inculet R, Nelems B (1992) Factors affecting cervical anastomotic leak and stricture formation following oesophagogastrectomy and gastric tube interposition. Am J Surg 163: 484–489

Fedele E, Del Prete M, Anselmo A (1996) Stapler. Perché quando come. Appunti sull'uso delle suturatrici meccaniche. Links, Rome

Feil W (1997) Schilddrüsenresektion mit UltraCision. Acta Chir Austr Suppl 130: 23

Feil W (1997) Sphinctererhaltende Rektumresektionen mit UltraCision. Acta Chir Austr Suppl 130: 80

Feil W (1997) UltraCision – Erste Erfahrungen in der offenen Chirurgie. Acta Chir Austr Suppl 130: 128

Feil W (1997) UltraCision – Erste Erfahrungen in der laparoskopischen Chirurgie. Acta Chir Austr Suppl 130: 130

Fok M, Wong J (1995) Cancer of the oesophagus and gastric cardia. Standard oesophagectomy and anastomotic technique. Ann Chir Gynaecol. 84: 179–183

Fowler DL (1996) Laparoscopic gastrectomy: five cases. Surg Laparosc Endosc 6: 98

Gabrelli F, Chiarelli M, Guttadauro A, Puana I, Faini G, Serbelloni M (1998) Considerazioni preliminari sulla muco-emorroidectomia con "stapler." UCP News Suppl 2: 6–7

Geis WP, Kim HC, McAffee PC, Kang JG, Brennan EJ (1996) Synergistic benefits of combined technologies in complex, minimally invasive surgical procedures. Surg Endosc 10: 1025

Gordon PH, Nivatvongs S (1999) Principles and practice of surgery for the colon, rectum, and anus. Quality Medical Publishing, St Louis

Gritsman JJ (1966) Mechanical suture by Soviet apparatus in gastric resection: use in 4,000 operations. Surgery 59: 663

Hampel N, Bodner DR, Persky L (1986) Ileal and jejunal conduit urinary diversion. Urol Clin North Am 13: 207

Heberer G, Schildberg FW, Sunder-Plassmann L, Vogt-Moykopf I (1991) Lunge und Mediastinum, 2. Aufl. Springer, Berlin Heidelberg New York

Iroatulam AJN, Banducci T, Vernillo R, Lorenzi M (1998) Transanal excision of mucosal rectal prolapse using a circular stapler. Colorectal Disease – Fort Lauderdale, Florida Pre-course Session II February 18, 1998

Kock NG (1969) Intra-abdominal reservoir in patients with permanent ileostomy: Preliminary observations on a procedure resulting in fecal continence in five ileostomy patients. Arch Surg 99: 223

Kock NF, et al (1982) Urinary diversion via a continent ileal reservoir: clinical result in 12 patients. J Urol 128: 469

Kohlstadt CM, Weber J, Prohm P (1999) Die Stapler-Hämorrhoidektomie. Eine neue Alternative zu den konventionellen Methoden. Zentralbl Chir 124: 238–243

Krasna MJ (1995) Left transthoracic oesophagectomy. Chest Surg Clin North Am 5: 543–554

Kremer K, Lierse W, Platzer W, Schreiber HW, Weller S (1989–1999) Chirurgische Operationslehre in 10 Bänden. Thieme, Stuttgart New York

Kremer K, Lierse W, Platzer W, Schreiber HW, Weller S (1995) Chirurgische Operationslehre, Bd. 7/2: Minimal-invasive Chirurgie. Thieme, Stuttgart New York

Lam TC, Fok M, Cheng SW, Wong J (1991) Anastomotic complications after oesophagectomy for cancer. A comparison of neck and chest anastomoses. World J Surg 15: 635–641

Lange V, Millot M, Dahsan H, Eilers D (1996) Das Ultraschallskalpell – erste Erfahrungen beim Einsatz in der laparoskopischen Chirurgie. Chirurg 67: 387

Laycock WS, Trus TL, Hunter JG (1996) New technology for the division of short gastric vessels during laparoscopic Nissen fundoplication. Surg Endosc 10: 71

Lippert H (1998) Praxis der Allgemein- und Viszeralchirurgie. Thieme, Stuttgart New York

Longo A (1998) Treatment of hemorrhoids disease by reduction of mucosa and hemorrhoidal prolapse with a circular suturing device: a new procedure. 6th World Congress of Endoscopic Surgery. Rome 1998, pp 777–784

Lozac'h P (1997) Intrathoracic anastomosis after oesophagectomy for cancer. J Chir Paris 134: 429–431

Lozac'h P, Topart P, Perramant M: Ivor Lewis procedure for epidermoid carcinoma of the oesophagus. A series of 264 patients.

MacKeigan JM, Cataldo PA (1993) Intestinal stomas. Principles, techniques, and management. Quality Medical Publishing, St Louis

Milito G, Cortese F, Casciani CU (1998) Surgical treatment of mucosal prolapse and haemorrhoids by stapler. 6th World Congress of Endoscopic Surgery. Rome 1998, pp 785–789

Moossa AR, Easter DW, Sonnenberg E, Casola G, Agostino H (1992) Laparoscopic injuries to the bilde duct. Ann Surg 215: 203

Orringer MB, Marshall B, Stirling MC (1993) Transhiatal oesophagectomy for benign and malignant disease. J Thorac Cardiovasc Surg 105: 265–276

Palazzini G (1988) Staple sutures in digestive tract surgery. Int Surg

Palazzini G, Tarroni D (1995) Errori di uomini e di macchine nell'uso delle suturatrici meccaniche in chirurgia colorettale. Colanna monografica S.I.C. 261–273

Palazzini G, Tarroni D, Monti M, Lippolis G, Vergine M, De Antoni E (1990) Le complianze delle suturatrici meccaniche nella chirurgia coloretalle: quando e perché. Atti 92° congresso SIC Roma 21–25/10/1990 volume 2: 5–26

Ravitch M, Febiger L (1991) Current practice of Surgical Stapling. Philadelphia

Ravitch MM, et al (1959) Experimental and clinical use of Soviet bronchus stapling instruments. Surgery 46: 97

Ravitch MM, Steichen FM (1972) Techniques of staple suturing in the gastrointestinal tract. Ann Surg 175: 815

Rehner M, Oestern H-J (1996) Chirurgische Facharztweiterbildung, Bd 1. Thieme, Stuttgart New York

Rothenberg SS (1996) Laparoscopic splenectomy using the Harmonic Scalpel. J Laparoendosc Surg 6: S61

Steichen FM, Ravitch MM (1973) Mechanical sutures in surgery. Br J Surg 70: 191

Steichen FM, Ravitch MM (1984) Stapling in surgery. Year Book Medical Publishing, Chicago

Sugarbaker DJ, Decamp MM (1993) Selecting the surgical approach to cancer of the oesophagus. Chest 103: 410S–414S

Swanstrom LL, Pennings JL (1995) Laparoscopic control of short gastric vessels. J Am Coll Surg 181: 347

Thüroff JW, Alken P, Hohenfellner R (1987) The Mainz pouch (mixed augmentation with ileum and cecum) for bladder augmentation and continent diversion. In: King LR et al (eds) Bladder reconstruction and continent urinary diversion. Year Book Medical Publishing, Chicago, p 252

Tilanus HW, Hop WC, Langenhorst BL, Van Lanschot JJ (1993) Oesophagectomy with or without thoracotomy. Is there any difference? J Thorac Cardiovasc Surg 105: 898–903

Traitment des hemorroides de stade 3 et 4 par la technique de Longo. Ann Chir Lyon (1999) 53: 245

Von Petz A (1924) Zur Technik der Magenresektion. Ein neuer Magen-Darmnähapparat. Zentralbl Chir 51, No. 5: 179–188

Retrieving Images from the CD-ROM

The attached CD-ROM, "Atlas of Surgical Stapling – Illustrations," contains all the images found in the book. You can copy these images into another program, or print them out.

Technical requirements

To retrieve these images you will need a personal computer with Windows 95 or higher, and at least:

- 133 MHz
- 32 MB RAM
- 4x CD-ROM
- VGA (640 × 480 pixels)
- 256 colors

Starting the Program

Insert CD into your CD-ROM drive. If Autostart is activated, the program will run automatically. Otherwise, double-click:

1. My Computer
2. CD-ROM
3. Atlas 32

Using the Program

Click Help for an explanation of all buttons and tabs.

Selection of illustrations

The Contents List tab will display a list of images and their page numbers.

You have two options:

1. Select an illustration by entering the page number, then pressing Enter on your keyboard. If the page contains more than one illustration, they will appear in alphabetical order.

2. Select an illustration by clicking the Index tab. Click on the desired image from the 20 that will be displayed successively. If the image you require does not appear on the selected Index page, click the Previous or Next button.

Printing and Exporting Illustrations

Click the Print Image or Export Image buttons.

Publication Data

Click the Publication Data button.

To Close the Program

Click Quit.